COMPENDIOUS
HOSPITAL MANAGEMENT

COMPENDIOUS
HOSPITAL MANAGEMENT

Dr. NILANJANA GHOSH

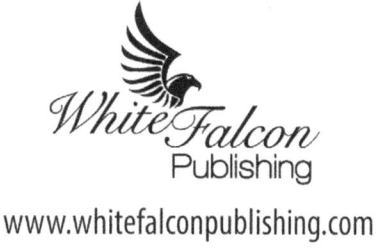

WhiteFalcon
Publishing

www.whitefalconpublishing.com

Compendious Hospital Management
Nilanjana Ghosh

www.whitefalconpublishing.com

ISBN - 978-1-63640-644-2

Contents

CHAPTER 1

Hospital Management Basics

Dr Mohammad Waseem Faraz Ansari

Assistant Professor, Department of Community Medicine,

ESIC Medical College & Hospital, Gulbarga, Karnataka

INTRODUCTION

Hospital management, also synonymised as hospital administration, has always been an integral part of the field of health management. Hospitals are a costly affair, contributing to a major chunk of the health service. Considering that the primary function of the hospital is to deliver comprehensive care to the community, it also serves to be the epitome of knowledge and skills to train all cadres of health workers viz., doctors, nurses and paramedics — while also serving as a centre for collateral continuous research. Hence, hospital management at its core, deals with administrative management as well as operational management to serve these purposes.

Weihrich and Koontz defined management as "the process of designing and maintaining an environment in which individuals, working together in groups, efficiently accomplish selected aims".[1]

Meanwhile, Mary Parker Follett defined management as "the art of getting things done through people". In all aspects, management means to bring forth the maximum output by an organisation as a result of optimum inputs from the individuals or groups. The organisation here is the hospital and the individuals and group accomplishing the aims and objectives are the health care workers.

The Two Facets of Hospital Management

Hospital management is a broad spectrum of managerial skills applied towards administrative management and operational management. The administrative management includes the policy framing and decision-making aspects, whereas the operational management deals with the implementation of these policies and decisions at the hospital. For a hospital to function optimally, both the administrative and the operational management has to be functioning as a coherent unit.

The System

Hospital management is a dynamic system which, in itself, is mainly composed of the following steps: the input, the process and the output (as evidenced in Figure 1).[2]

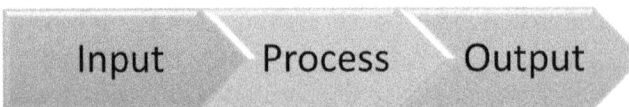

Figure 1: The steps of health management system

Although the system translates into these three important steps, the whole phenomenon is never complete without rendering the expected outcomes and also the feedback which paves the way for regulating and improving the process of management (as depicted in Figure 2).

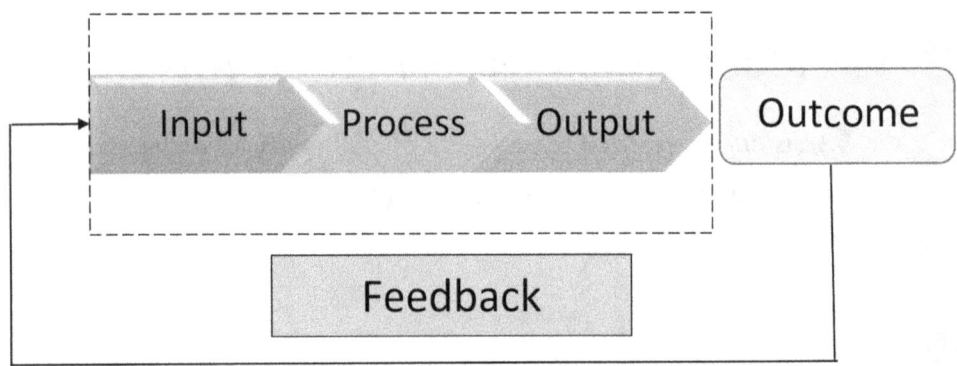

Figure 2: The steps of health management system with outcome and feedback

As far as the health management is concerned, the steps of the process can be enlisted in terms of the investment and the outcome expected. This is evidenced in the following table:

Input/Resources	Process	Output	Outcome
Manpower	Planning	No of lives saved	Reduced morbidity
Materials	Organising	No of diseases prevented	Reduced mortality
Money	Coordinating	No of patients treated	Reduced disability
Time	Executing	No of patients rehabilitated	Comprehensive health care delivery to the community

The Manager

The manager is the person who is carrying out all the processes of the management through his position. For the optimum output, the following functions have to be performed with utmost diligence and meticulous coordination.[3]

1. **Planner:** The manager has to be a planner of the process at both micro and macro levels. The policy making, the strategy and its implementation have to be planned by the manager.
2. **Organiser:** The plan, once laid, must be carried through to success on the shoulders of an exceptional organiser of resources.
3. **Director:** The manager directs the working of each member of the team, defines their roles and responsibilities, monitors their working pattern and improves their efforts.

4. **Staffer:** It is the manager who ensures the staff placement, recruitment and delegation of appropriate staff at their respective positions.

5. **Coordinator:** The manager must regulate that the organisation is functioning in congruence by ensuring coordination of each staff to promote high output via integrated work efforts.

6. **Reviewer:** The functioning of the management and the performance of the team must be regulated from time to time by reviewing their performance, critiquing and improving the organised efforts.

7. **Budgeter:** The manager must draw a budgeting draft for smooth functioning of the hospital as well as analyse things on the basis of cost effectiveness and benefit.

8. **Facilitator:** The manager must facilitate the whole system from the conceptual framework to the implementation of the plan and reviewing of the process, so that the members of the team and, in fact, the whole process is existing smoothly and functioning effectively.

9. **Decision Maker:** The manager must be a decision maker at any given point of time —especially in times of crisis as the functioning of the team and allocation of the resources is dependent on the decisions of the strategy maker.

10. **Strategist:** The manager must be a good strategy maker to plan in such a manner that the desired goal is achieved.

Skills of Hospital Administrator

The role of a hospital administrator is to facilitate the principles of management by executing the managerial functions through a multifaceted approach; therefore, this requires certain skills. The skills required at different levels of management viz. top, middle and lower levels are not proportionately similar.

1. **Coordination Skills:** Coordination skills are quintessential at any level of management to ensure that the team is functioning as a unit towards the desired objectives, though it finds its application at higher level of management.

2. **Computer Skills:** The health information system has to be updated and this requires computer skills on the part of any administrator; essentially, they should know how different softwares perform. The computer skills are directly proportional to the productivity.

3. **Conceptual Skills:** The conceptual skills in health management are primarily at the higher tiers of managerial position where the functioning of the system has to be in alignment of the desired vision.

4. **Decision Making Skills:** To have various options available and to decide among them the best as per the situation is an important trait of a manager not only in normal functioning but especially during crises and crucial times.

5. **Analytical Skills:** The manager must be able to analyse a situation to increase the productivity so as to make the hospital highly efficient, identify the shortcomings, strengthen the strengths and implement new reforms which will ensure that the hospital runs with optimum efficiency at regular intervals.

6. **Human Relation Skills:** No hospital can function effectively without its manager possessing good human relations skills. Medical humanities is a wider horizon and every hospital administrator need to be good at human relations because in a bigger picture, saidmanagement has to work with the cooperation of the people to be able to fulfil its role towards the community.

7. **Communication Skills:** The manager must be an excellent communicator at every level of the hospital management system. Communication encompasses verbal and non-verbal communication skills, the body language, and the dos and don'ts of ideal communication which ensure that the message is conveyed efficiently.

8. **Technical Skills:** Though the technical skills find their application more towards the lower levels of health management system, it is not at all ignored as the health administrator should be well versed with the technical capabilities both of themselves and the team they are managing so that at times when required, they can prove themselves to be a team member with exceptional proficiency in the psychomotor domain.

References

1. Harold Koontz, et al. *Essentials of Management* (5th edition). McGraw-Hill International Edition, 1990.
2. Joshi DC. *Hospital Administration* (1st edition). Jaypee Brothers, 2009.
3. PV Sathe, PP Doke. *Epidemiology and Management for Healthcare* (5th edition). Vora Medical Publishers, 2018.

CHAPTER 2
Organisational Behavior

Dr Neeraj Gour

Professor, Department of Community Medicine
SHKM Govt. Medical college, Nuh, Haryana

Dr Meenakshi Chaudhary

Consultant Pathologist, Haryana

INTRODUCTION

Organisational Behavior (OB) is usually defined as the understanding, prediction and management of human behaviour both individually or in a group that occur within an organisation. When we are working in an organisation, it is very much pertinent to understand others' behaviour as well as make others understand ours. In a bid to establish and maintain a healthy working environment, we need to adapt to the environment and understand the goals we need to achieve. This can be accomplished with best outcomes if we understand the importance of organisational behaviour.

Salient Points on the Importance of OB

- It helps in explaining the interpersonal relationships employees share with each other as well as with their higher and lower subordinates.
- The prediction of individual behaviour can be studied in detail.
- It balances the cordial relationship in an organisation by maintaining effective communication.
- It assists in most fruitful decision making.
- It helps managers to encourage and motivate their subordinates.
- Any change within the organisation can be made easier.
- It helps in predicting human behaviour and their application to achieve organisational goals.
- It helps in making the organisation more effective and efficient.

Organisational behaviour usually starts with patterns of human behaviour and end at the point og the performance of an organisation.

Determinants of Organisational Behaviour

There are three major determinants of organisational behaviour which determine the working environment of that organisation.

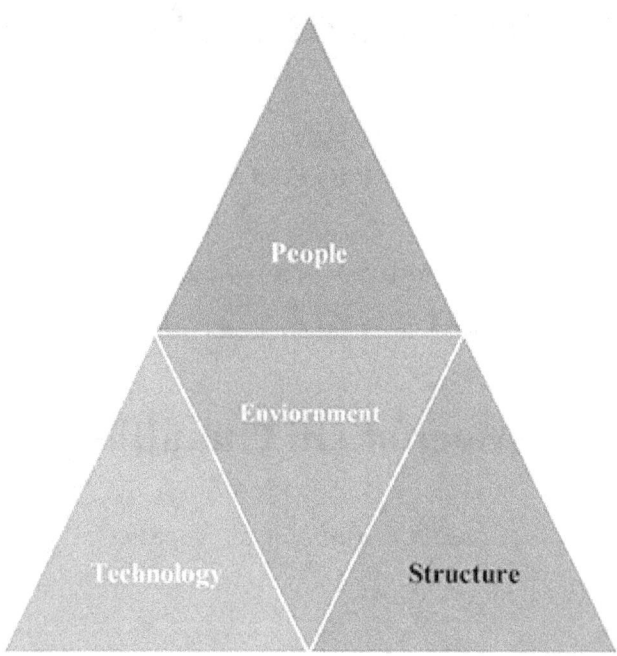

People

Any organisation consists of people with different traits, personality, skills, qualities, interests, background, beliefs, values and intelligence. To ensure and maintain a healthy environment, all the employees should be treated equally and be judged according to their work and other aspects that affect the firm

Organisational Structure

Structure is the layout design of an organisation. It is the establishment and arrangement of relationships and strategies according to the organisational goal and targets.

Technology

Technology is defined as the implementation of scientific knowledge for practical use. It also provides resources needed by the people that influence their work and task performance to move in the right and appropriate direction.

Environment

All organisations function within a given internal and external environment. Internal environment can be defined as the conditions, factors, and elements within an organisation that influence the activities and choices made by the same, and especially the behaviour of the employees. External environment, meanwhile, can be defined as outside factors that affect the organisation's ability to work. Some examples of internal environment include employee morale, culture changes, financial changes or issues, and some examples of external environment include political factors, changes to the economy and the organisation itself.

Concepts of Organisational Behaviour	
Nature of People	**Nature of Organisation**
Individual Difference Perception A whole person Motivated behaviour Value of person	Social system (formal and informal) Mutual interest Ethics

Models of Organisational Behaviour

There are four different types of models of organisational behaviour. The salient points of each model are enumerated in the following table:

Autocratic Model	**Custodial Model**
Power with a managerial orientation of authority Obedience and discipline Dependence on their boss Performance result is less People are easily frustrated, and there is insecurity and dependency on the superiors	Economic resources with a managerial orientation of money Employees are oriented towards security and benefits Dependence on the organisation The approach directs one to depend on firm rather than on manager or boss Employees are satisfied but not strongly encouraged
Supportive Model	**Collegial Model**
Leadership with a managerial orientation of support Employees oriented towards their job performance and participation Dependence on leadership Employees feel a sense of participation	Partnership with a managerial orientation of teamwork Responsible behaviour and self-discipline Self-actualisation and moderate zeal Team work approach is adapted • Sense of "accept" and "respect" is seen

Theories of Organisational Behaviour

There are many theories propounded for organisational behaviour; some of them are elaborated below with their salient points.

Sigmund Freud's Psychoanalytic Theory

This theory is based on the belief that an individual is encouraged more by unforeseen forces than the conscious and logical thought. This is based on three attributes: id, ego and superego.

Sheldon's Physiognomy Theory

This theory was proposed by William Sheldon. It focuses upon personalities by classifying individuals into convenient categories based on their body shapes. They are:

- Endomorphs
- Mesomorphs
- Ectomorphs

Erikson's Theory

This theory states that personality is groomed throughout lifetime.

Maslow's Hierarchy of Needs Theory

This theory was propounded in a bid to answer the question "What motivates an individual?" Each second need comes to force when the first need is satisfied altogether. These needs follow a particular order, starting from physiological needs and going on to safety needs, social needs, esteem and self-actualisation.

Theory X and Theory Y

Theory X: This theory believes that employees are naturally unmotivated and dislike working, and this encourages an authoritarian style of management.

Theory Y: This theory explains a participative style of management, that is distributive in nature. It states that employees are happy to work, self-motivated and creative, and enjoy working with greater responsibility and accountability.

Behavioural Theory

This theory explains the effectiveness of leadership. As per this theory, leadership has two qualities i.e., initiating structure and consideration. These varieties of qualities are tested with higher and lower levels with proper intersection of each other.

Contingency Theory

This theory was propounded by Paul Hersey and Ken Blanchard, and they believe that the effectiveness of a leader is dependent on the action or readiness of his followers. It depends on interaction of task and relationship behaviour between leader and the leader's subordinates.

Group Decision-making

Group decision-making, usually known as collaborative decision-making, is a situation that emerges when individuals collectively make a choice from the alternatives options before them.

There are many group decision-making theories that are available in literature; some of them are mentioned below:

Brainstorming	1. Five and ten in number 2. Free association 3. Main focus is on generation of ideas and not on evaluation of these ideas 4. More ideas can be originated 5. Very effective when the problem is comparatively precise and simply defined
1. Similar to brainstorming except that this approach is more structured 2. Members do not communicate well with each other so that strong personality domination is evaded 3. Group coordinator either collects the written ideas or writes them on a large blackboard and discusses them 4. Highest cumulative ranking idea is selected as the final solution	**Nominal Group Thinking**
Didactic Interaction	1. Applicable only in certain situations 2. Type of problem should be such that it generates output in the form of yes or no
1. Improvised version of the nominal group technique 2. Opinions of experts physically distant from each other and unknown to each other 3. Process of sending questionnaires, results and review until we reach a final decision with agreement.	**Delphi Technique**

Points to Remember

1. Organisational behaviour is one of the backbones of health care management.

2. It is a management science which mainly focuses on people, structure, environment and technology of organisation in a bid to increase the productivity of same and achieve the desired outcomes.

3. There are many theories of organisational behaviour, i.e. personality theories, leadership theories, behavioural theories, etc. Managers can pick whichever of these is best suited for their organisation.

4. There are mainly four models of organisational behaviour, namely autocratic, collegial, supportive and custodial model. Any one of them may be adopted by managers or a contingency approach may also be followed depending upon the situation and organisation.

Bibliography & Suggested Readings:

1. JM Ivancevich, MT Matteson, R Konopask. *Organizational Behavior and Management.*

2. https://www.iedunote.com/forces-affecting-organizational-behavior.

3. J Wood, R Zeffane, M Fromholtz, R Wiesner, RR Morrison, A Factor, T McKeown. *Organisational Behaviour: Core Concepts and Applications*. John Wiley & Sons Australia, Ltd., 2019.

4. PS Rao. *Organisational Behaviour*. Himalaya Publishing House, 2010.

5. https://www.semanticscholar.org/paper/Comparison-Of-The-Models-Of-Organizational-A-Review-Wibo wo/1e09f27e911752f09dde80f49f2f28bdea7c4073.

6. N Singh. *Organisational Behaviour: Concepts, Theory and Practices: Managing People and Organisations in the 21st Century*. Deep and Deep Publications, 2001.

7. https://www.slideshare.net/RINKUV/techniques-of-group-decision-making.

CHAPTER 3

Communications in Health Management

Dr. Rabbanie Tariq

Lifestyle Medicine Physician & Public Health Specialist

Joint Secretary, Indian Society of Lifestyle Medicine

HEALTH AND COMMUNICATION

The communication in health management involves the utilization of communication strategies to influence individual and community knowledge, attitudes and practices (KAP) with respect to health and general population. These gaps are more visible among (a) marginalized strata like those with low literacy, limited English proficiency or low socioeconomic status, and low literacy (b) stigmatized groups like those with HIV-AIDS, obesity, or mental conditions, and (c) minority populations and refugees. Poor communication incorporates a strongly negative impact on outcomes of diseases like (a) Non-Communicable/lifestyle diseases including diabetes and hypertension, (b) acute illnesses, including pain control, morbidity following surgery, and length of hospital stay, and (c) mental illnesses like depression and schizophrenia. Improvements in communication in healthcare settings, invariably result in better health outcomes. Furthermore, these changes may contribute to greater equity in health and healthcare for racial, ethnic, socioeconomic, educational and minority populations. Better communication can cause improvements in prevention, motivation for behavior change, and adherence to treatment.

Communication in explicit terms refers to the transmission or exchange of any reasonably information among those who are communicating. Communication serves the needs of: a) starting actions, b) informing needs c) exchanging ideas, attitudes, beliefs & information d) engendering understanding, e) establishing and maintaining relations. Communication, thus, plays an integral role within the delivery of healthcare and therefore the promotion of health, health communication encompasses the study and use of communication strategies to influence individual and community decisions that enhance health. It acts a bridge between knowledge gap and health promotion, moreover as education.

Trends and Their Effects on Communication

Globally, population has experienced fluctuating demographic trends during the last five decades. Demographically, these trends are important in this they need contributed to the changing composition of the world population; this, in turn, has influenced the morbidity profile of population existed over time.

Indeed, the demographic transformation and longevity of the Indian population are one of the dire needs to be addressed by the healthcare system.

Throughout recorded history, acute health conditions have constituted the main health threat and therefore the leading causes of death for any population. At the start of the 20th century, among the topmost causes of mortality were infectious diseases because the deathrate for the South Asian population declined during the late twentieth century and lifespan began increase, a major change materialized in the morbidity and mortality profile of the population (1). During the late twentieth century, the changing demographic profile led to a shift from acute conditions to lifestyle diseases because the predominant variety of pathological state. Improved living conditions, better nutrition, sedentary lifestyle and better standards of living, amid advances in bioscience, reduced or eliminated the burden of acute disease conditions. The gap was filled up, however, by the emergence of lifestyle diseases - the leading health issues and leading causes of death. The elderly population that resulted from these developments was now full of Non-communicable diseases, yet as numerous conditions that reflected the lifestyles characterizing the population within the half of that century.

An Account of Inception of Health Communication

The emergence of health as a crucial personal concern and also the ascendancy of healthcare as a significant institution within the middle of the 20th century among developed countries were major factors in evolving the sphere of health communication. The conceptualization of "health" as valuable entity globally represented a landmark development in arising of healthcare institution. Earlier to World War II health was generally not recognized in world but was vaguely tied in with other notions of well-being. After the war personal health became a growing concern, and therefore the adequate provision of health services became a very important issue within the mind of the overall public. By the last third of the 20th century, health had become of prime importance with policy makers. Once health became established as a worth, it had been a brief step to establishing a proper healthcare system because the institutional means for achieving that value. An environment was created that encouraged the emergence of a robust institution that supported many other contemporary moral values. within the half of the 20th century emerging concepts of progression of life for youth, their beauty and self-actualization, which further contributed to an expansion of the role of healthcare. the power of the nascent healthcare system to handle emerging health indicators and garner support from the economic, political, and academic institutions assured the ascendancy of this new institutional form.

Initial Interventions of Health Communication

As medicine evolved in developed countries, health communication was poorly developed. The sphere of communication wasn't recognized as a definite discipline and far was considered to be relevant to arena of "common sense". To be sure, there have been announcements of quarantine and other alerts/communications associated with infectious diseases and related outbreaks. But the sensible application of health communication had not achieved its target. The religion healers—who could have been anyone - communicated the contents, techniques and used natural materials for the management of disease and injury. Intergenerational word of mouth was critical for passing on of the accumulated knowledge of traditional medicine to subsequent generations. In early twentieth century, few people had the privilege to use doctors. Availability & Accessibility was limited and to some extent that continues even today. There was no dominant medical supporting evidence and, in a very democratic society, any man's medicine was pretty much as good as the next one's. In actually, those that passed for "doctors" in those days didn't have much within the way of information, tools, or skills when it came to most of the health conditions that existed during those days. The one brilliant tool they did have, however, was their communication skills—their bedside mannerisms, that they developed during the course of their careers. Given the actual fact that nobody had the required skills to cure most diseases, medical historians report that those with effective communication skills had the most effective chance of affecting a cure. Hitherto, even today we recognize the importance of a healing environment and therefore the impact that communication can wear the course of an illness.

Models of the Evolution of Health Communication

Evolving Medical Models

The scientific theory evolution with the concurrent emergence of the allopathic belief models led to acceleration to healthcare which proved to be a blessing in disguise. While the contribution of scientific medicine to the conquest of disease may be overstated (McKinley and McKinley, 1977), a critical approach to the management of illness was created that contributed to raising the health status for people and communities. As it became more science based, it became increasingly reductionist, with all health problems pursued all the way down to rock bottom level—from the person to the body system to the organ to the cellular structure. With each successive step, the patient as a human being receded further into the background. The direct implication of this development was the demeaning of the importance of communication towards patients/clients manner was relegated to the medical archives, since the solution to the matter was to be found under the microscopic evaluations and not within the patient. While some physicians developed a good manner, organized medicine came to determine this as an unnecessary skill. During the "golden age" of medication within the developed countries—the 1960s and 70s—health communication was further pushed to the corner. As medicine became more scientific, the importance of detached objectivity came to the force. Instead of coming to know the totality of the patient, physicians were now trained to stay distant and uninvolved, lest personal feelings interfere with the march of medical progress. Since it a was absolutely impossible to totally avoid communication with patients and/or their families, the conversation of physicians became stuffed with medical jargon. Their new-found knowledge base allowed them to demonstrate the extent of skill they possessed and created a transparent separation between the learned practitioner and also the ignorant patient. Thus, physicians came to use scientific terminology that they were reluctant to elucidate to patients. Further, the asymmetric nature of the link discouraged questions on the part of patients—lest they seem to question the pronouncements of the great doctor. These developments contributed to a decline within the quality of doctor-patient interaction and thus reduction in patient satisfaction.

Patient Awareness Generation

A reaction to the existing approach after 1970s started with regard to dying doctor-patient relationships which was known as the "patient education movement". Earlier, patients were woefully unaware of the character of health and illness and unable to contribute to their health status in a meaningful way. The causes for this fall of communication are related primarily to the healthcare system and particularly on the physicians. Observers cited the deliberate efforts on the part of physicians to hamper communication, deter the transfer of information, and obscure things within the mind of the patient. Health care practitioners justified their lapses in communication on the grounds that patients were unable to intelligently speak about their problems, heavy rush of patient load, a claim that was refuted by research indicating reasonable knowledge of patients, even patients considered to be disadvantaged. Although, the disturbed doctor- patient ratio continues to be a downgrading factor for health communication.

Health Communication Users

There are various potential audiences for health communication activities Differences within the characteristics of people (e.g., patients, caregivers), social groups (e.g., staff), and communities as audiences are reviewed. Health professionals and facilities are major consumers of products and services within the healthcare arena. The main terms used in health communication audiences are described below.

Clients: A client could be sort of customer that consumes services instead of goods. A client interaction implies personal (rather than impersonal) repo building and an on-going relationship (rather than an episodic one). Professionals typically have clients while retailers, as an example, would have customers or purchasers.

Customers: The "customer" is usually thought of in healthcare a purchaser of service. While a patient could also be a customer of goods and services, it's often the case that the end-user (e.g., the patient) might not be the customer. Some other person may make the acquisition on behalf of the patient, and treatment decisions is also made by someone apart from the patient. For this reason, hospitals and other complex healthcare organizations are likely to serve a variety of consumers. These may include patients, staff physicians, health plans, employers and other personnel who may purchase goods or services from the organization.

Consumers: "Consumer" is any person or organization who's a possible purchaser of a healthcare service. Theoretically, most are a possible consumer of health services, and market research often targets the general public at large. The healthcare consumer is usually the end-user of service but might not necessarily be the purchaser.

Patients: The term "patient" implies someone who has been admitted into the formal system of healthcare. Technically, a symptomatic individual doesn't become a patient until a physician officially designates the individual intrinsically, whether or not he has consumed over-the-counter drugs or taken other measures for self-care. Under this scenario, a person remains a patient until he's discharged from medical aid. Sometimes, mental therapists are likely to visit the people they supply services to as "clients" instead of "patients" for establishing a more robust repo with the person.

End-users: In healthcare, the end-user is sometimes a patient who is the direct recipient of a health service or the eventual consumer of a health product or over the- counter drug.

References

National Cancer Institute. (2003). Making health communication work. Washington: federal government Printing Office.

Health Communication and its Influence Behavior Related to Health

Relevant theories formulated to clarify health behavior are presented and their relevance to health communication are discussed below:

Health Behavior Models:

There are a series of models that are developed geared to the individual, the group and also the community (National Cancer Institute, 2003). Although there's no generally accepted model, the foremost important ones are described below.

Level of Individuality: One set of models of health behavior focuses on the individual level and considers how individuals make decisions with relation to health behavior. Effective communication under these styles of models requires an in-depth understanding of individual traits and attributes.

Behavioral Intentions: Studies of behavioral intentions suggest that the likelihood of intended audiences' adopting a desired behavior is predicted by assessing (and subsequently trying to alter or influence) their attitudes toward and perceptions of advantages of the behavior. Therefore, a crucial step toward influencing behavior may be a preliminary assessment of the stage of behavior change the intended audience attitudes.

Stages of Behavior Change: The essential procedure of the stages-of-behavior change is that behavior change could be a dynamic process and not static. Further, individuals are considered to be at varying levels of motivation or readiness to alter their behaviors. The extent to which individuals are tuned in to change will rely upon their level of acceptability to change. Knowing an individual's active stage allows communicators to line realistic & achievable program goals. It's possible to customize messages, strategies, and programs to the acceptable stage.

Six distinct stages are identified within the stages-of-change construct: 1. Precontemplation 2. Contemplation 3. Preparation 4. Action 5. Maintenance 6. Relapse. It's important to notice that this is often a circular, not a linear, model. Individuals can enter or exit at any time and re-enter any phase through the model.

(a) Health Belief Model:

The health belief model (HBM) was originally designed to clarify why people failed to participate in programs to forestall or detect diseases. The core components of the HBM include:

Perceived susceptibility—the subjective perception of risk of developing a specific health condition
Perceived severity—feelings about the seriousness of the results of developing a selected unhealthiness
Perceived benefits—beliefs about the effectiveness of assorted actions which may reduce susceptibility and severity
Perceived barriers—potential negative aspects of taking specific actions
Cues to action—bodily or environmental events that trigger action

More recently, the HBM has been amended to incorporate the notion of self-efficacy as another predictor of health behaviors, especially more complex ones during which lifestyle changes must be maintained over time.

(b) Consumer Information Model

Information may be a common tool for health education and is usually a necessary foundation for health decisions. The conveyance of knowledge can increase or decrease people's anxiety, considering their information preferences and also the amount and sort of data they're given. Illness and its treatments can interfere with information science. By understanding the key concepts and processes of CIP, health educators can examine why people use or fail to use health information and subsequently design simpler communication strategies. CIP theory reflects a mixture of rational and motivational ideas.

Level of Interpersonal connections:

Another form of model posits that behavior could be a function of the influence of interpersonal relationships within which the individual is involved. These relationships provide clues—if not outright direction—for behavior.

(a) Social Cognitive Theory:

Social cognitive theory (SCT) explains behavior in terms of triadic reciprocity during which behavior, cognitive and other interpersonal factors, and environmental events all operate as interacting determinants of one another. SCT describes behavior as dynamically determined and fluid, influenced by both personal factors and also the environment. Changes in any of those three factors are hypothesized to engender changes within the others. SCT views the environment as not just a variable that reinforces or punishes behaviors, but one that also provides a milieu during which a person can watch the actions of others and learn the results of these behaviors. Processes governing observational learning include:

Attention—gaining and maintaining attention
Retention—being remembered
Reproduction—reproducing the observed behavior
Motivation—being stimulated to provide the behavior
Organization/Community/Societal Level:

A third sort of model operates at the more macro levels of organization, community and society. Communication activities at these levels is also geared to influencing organizational change, modifying the environment of the community, or influencing public policy. Given this, communication efforts under this model are likely to require a range of forms and be particularly complex.

(b) Organizational Change Theory:

Organizations represent complex social systems composed of the many components. Organizational change can best be promoted by performing at multiple levels within the organization. Understanding organizational change is very important for establishing policies and environments that support healthy practices and make the capacity to unravel new problems. While there are many theories of organization behavior, two are especially of interest to us here: stage theory and organizational development (OD) theory.

Stage theory is predicated on the thought that organizations suffer a series of steps or stages as they alter. Strategies to push change is matched to varied points within the process of change. An abbreviated version of stage theory involves four stages: Problem definition, Initiation of action, Implementation, Institutionalization. A typical OD strategy involves process consultation, within which an outdoor specialist helps identify problems and facilitates the design of change in strategies (including communication approaches). Stage theory and OD theory have the best potential to provide health-enhancing change in organizations after they are combined. That is, OD strategies may be used at various stages as they're warranted.

(c) Community Organization Theory:

Community organization theory has its origin in theories of social networks and support. It emphasizes active participation in developing communities that may better evaluate and solve health and social problems. Community organization is that the process by which communities identify problems, mobilize resources, and develop and implement plans for reaching specified goals. Some approaches to community change include:

Locality development (also called community development) uses a wider scale of individuals within the community to spot and solve its own problems. It stresses consensus development, capacity building, and a powerful task orientation; outside practitioners help to coordinate and enable the community to successfully address its concerns.

Social planning uses tasks and goals, and addresses substantive problem solving, with expert practitioners providing technical assistance to learn community members.

Social action helps in problem-solving ability of the community and to attain concrete changes to redress social injustice that's identified by a disadvantaged or oppressed group. Although community organization theory doesn't use one unified model, several key concepts are central to the varied approaches. the method of empowerment is meant to stimulate problem solving and activate community members. Community competence is an approximate community-level equivalent of self-efficacy plus behavioral capability, which involves the arrogance and skills to resolve problems effectively. Participation and relevance involve citizen enlightenment and a collective sense of readiness to improve.

Diffusion of Innovations: Diffusion of innovations theory addresses how new ideas, products, and social knowledge/practices spread within a community or from one society to a different one. The challenge of diffusion requires a *modus operandi* that differ from those focused solely on individuals or small groups. This approach requires attention to the innovation (a new idea, product, practice, or technology) further on communication channels and social systems (networks with members, norms, and social structures).

Nature of Communication

"Communication" involves the transfer of data from sender to receiver, for the aim of accelerating the receiver's information status, enabling him to hold out tasks, or influencing his attitudes and behavior. The "information" transferred refers to the conceptual representation of aspects of a universe within the variety of a message that may be encoded, transcripted and transmitted. Health communication will be used to: Initiate actions, ascertain needs and requirements, Exchange information, ideas, attitudes or beliefs, establish understanding, Establish and maintain relations. The extent to which a health communication effort serves these purposes depends on the character of the initiative and therefore the goals that are being pursued.

Communication Sources:

Communication is generated by an array of sources, and therefore the source is commonly critical to the acceptability of the message. Sources are often grouped into some major categories and therefore the ones most relevant to healthcare are discussed below.

Formal Sources:

Formal sources of health information include those entities that communicate with consumers as a part of their job. However, in healthcare with its technical dimension, physicians and other providers constitute a primary source of health information. All healthcare organizations offer some kind of information and, whether or not within the information business, most healthcare organizations must make referrals, conveying information within the process.

Impersonal Sources:

As mass media became pervasive, an increasing proportion of the population came to receive its information— on healthcare and other topics— from newspapers, magazines, radio and tv. These modes of knowledge transfer are the hallmark of recent society, with now emerging as more pivotal to mass media. Health could be a favorite topic of traditional media, and cable television has served to multiply the opportunities for health and healthcare programming. Popular books on healthcare have also become a significant source of knowledge on the subject regardless of the source, the effectiveness of a message depends to an oversized extent on the audience's perception of the source. "Perception" is critical since perceptions instead of reality may determine the style during which the message is received. The communicator's job is to regulate and determine the audience's perceptions. Students of communication have identified several dimensions of source credibility (O'Keefe, 1990), listed here so as of their importance:

1. Competence
2. Trustworthiness
3. Goodwill
4. Idealism
5. Similarity

Components of Communication:

Communication involves variety of components each of which is critical for a successful communication effort. the foremost components of the communication process are discussed below.

Context:

The context or environment is that the situation within which the communication occurs and includes the physical context, social context, number of individuals involved, relationship of participants, surrounding events, culture, rituals, and noise. The physical context is that the place during which the communication actually occurs. This might be within the receiver's home, workplace, physician's office, or other physical settings. The context would be quite different, as an example, for preachers delivering a sermon from a pulpit, on the road corner, or over a Television channel. The temperature, the time of day, nearby audience, and activities running in parallel all contribute to the establishment of a context. The social context represents a significant influence on communication. The context could also be a bunch of friends, work associates, or strangers. The context could also be familiar or strange. The context for the transmission of health information is a vital consideration. The identical information conveyed by the physician in his/her office, at work, from a friend, or via the web will have different degrees of impact. Some contexts are clearly more conducive to the transfer of health-related information than others.

Message:

Within the communication field, a message represents information that's sent from a source to a receiver. The message includes a thought or idea communicated briefly in a plain or secret language prepared in a very form suitable for transmission by different modes of communication. The message is a response, set of instructions, or recommendations that help accomplish the aim of the communication process. Health communicators must determine what information is to be provided, the design and tone during which it's presented, and what the message must ultimately convey. If the message doesn't resonate with the audience, the communication effort is probably going to fail.

Channels:

Communication occurs through a particular channel or channels. Channels also are remarked because the medium, hence references to "mass media" or to "the media" as a collective term for journalists working in any style of mass media. The channel determines the means within which the communication is delivered and received. Channels differ from one another in terms of attributes, attention getting, and volume of knowledge conveyed, among other factors. A book, for instance, has more credibility than television. More information are often communicated through a news article than a television newscast. In contrast to this, television has live pictures that make the communication more engaging. Each style of channel has merits and demerits. Factors to be considered in selecting a channel (and inquiries to be asked) include:

The intended audience(s)
Compatibility with the message
Channel reach
Cost and accessibility
Activities and materials:

Timing:

Timing will be thought of during a kind of ways. in an exceedingly mechanical sense, timing could visit the day of the week or time of the day at which communication occurs. It could also talk to the frequency of exposures established. Radio and tv advertising is carefully planned to require advantage of the habits of listeners or viewers, and knowledge is accessible on the timing that's appropriate for various target audiences. Timing can also sit down with the state of readiness on the part of the target vis-`a-vis the message that's being conveyed. Different audiences are amenable to the receipt of knowledge at different times, not in terms of indication but in terms of their current situation.

The Communication Process

A number of scientists in health communication have adopted one in all the models of communication for healthcare. While Communication experts focuses on marketing communication, this model may be readily applied to health communication. An understanding of every of those nine components is vital for effective communication.

1. The sender: is the entity sending the message to a different entity. Also known as the communicator or the source, the sender can be a company or spokesperson or any source of information.
2. The message refers to the amalgam of symbols and words that the sender wishes to transmit to the receiver. This indicates the content that the sender wants to convey. This means the "what" of communication process.
3. Encoding refers to the method of translating the desirable messaged to be transmitted into symbolic form (words, signs, sounds, etc.). At this stage, an idea is converted into something transmittable.
4. The channel are the means accustomed to propagate a marketing message from sender to receiver. This means the "how" of the method or what connects the sender to the receiver.
5. The receiver is that the party who receives the message, also called the audience or the destination. it's the receiver toward whom the communication effort is directed.
6. Decoding refers to the method dole out by the receiver when he converts the "symbols" transmitted by the sender into a form that produces sense to him. This process assumes that the receiver is using the identical basis for decoding that the sender used for encoding.
7. The response refers to the reaction of the receiver to the message. this can be the purpose at which the effect of the message is gauged, and relates to the meaning that the receiver attaches thereto.

8. Feedback refers to the aspect of the receiver's response that the receiver communicates back to the sender. the kind of feedback will rely upon the channel, and also the effectiveness of the trouble caused is gauged in terms of the feedback.

9. Noise refers to any factor that forestalls the decoding of a message by the receiver within the way intended by the sender. Noise are often generated by anyone within the communication process i.e., sender, the receiver, the message, the channel, the environment.

Barriers to Communication

The communication process may be inhibited by any number of things that may influence this process which can include selective attention on the part of the receiver, selective distortion on the part of the receiver, selective recall whereby the receiver only absorbs a part of the message, and message rehearsal whereby the receiver is reminded by the message of related issues that tend to distract the receiver from the purpose of the message. Any of the aspects of communication discussed above can have barriers related to them. These include the source of the data, context, message, channel and/or timing. a number of the barriers are discussed below.

Conflicting Messages: Messages that cause a conflict in perception for audience may lead to incomplete communication. as an example, if someone constantly uses jargon or slang to speak with someone from another country who has never heard such expressions, mixed messages are absolute to result. Another example of conflicting messages may well be if a supervisor requests a report immediately without giving the report writer enough time to collect the right information.

Information Overload: really, people don't concentrate to all or any communications they receive but selectively attend to and purposefully search out information. A received message containing an excessive amount of information is probably going to make a barrier to effective communication. If information is coming too fast and furious, people tend to place up barriers since the quantity of knowledge is coming so fast that it becomes difficult to interpret the data. this can be an innate trait of groups of people and may be seen in a baby that miraculously falls asleep within the face of intrusive attention. If a subject has 25 salient points, it's going to be possible to only communicate two or three of them at one time; otherwise the receiver is overwhelmed by the avalanche of data.

Transmission Barriers: Things that get within the way of message transmission are sometimes called "noise." Communication is also difficult thanks to noise and associated problems. a nasty cell phone line or a loud restaurant can inhibit communication.

Channel Barriers: the selection of channel is critical for effective communication and, if a sender chooses an inappropriate channel of communication, insurmountable barriers could also be imposed. Detailed instructions presented over the phone, for instance, could also be frustrating for both communicators. Some consumers are also so immune to direct (read "junk") mail, that they refuse to handle any organization that sends them unsolicited communication within the mail. The credibility (or lack thereof) of a channel will depend on the extent to which the message is appropriate to the receiver.

Literacy Levels: The literacy level of any audience must be taken into consideration. Health literacy is defined because the ability to read, understand, and act on health information. People of any age, income, race, or background can find it challenging to grasp health information. Low health literacy has been identified as a significant barrier to health communication, yet presenting material to well-educated audiences that's well below their level of comprehension may have a negative affect on the communication process. The health literacy problem involves more of a problem of understanding medical information instead of one amongst access to information. Medical information is becoming increasingly complex and, only too frequently, physicians don't explain this information in layperson's terms, or in an exceedingly way that patients can understand. Physicians are under increasing time pressure in today's clinical setting, and that they might not even remember when patients don't understand medical information or instructions. If patients don't understand medication and self-care instructions, a vital a part of their treatment is missing, which can then have an adverse effect on their clinical outcomes.

Social and Cultural Barriers: Effective communication with people of various cultures is particularly challenging. Cultures provide people with ways of seeing, hearing, and interpreting the planet. Thus the identical words can mean various things to people from different cultures, even once they talk the "same" language. When the languages are different, and translation should be tough to communicate, the potential for misunderstandings increases. Communication Experts define 3 ways within which culture interferes with effective cross-cultural understanding. *First* is what they call as "cognitive constraints." These are the frames of reference or universal views that provide an idea that each one new information is compared to or inserted into. This framework facilities one's interpretation of the data that's transmitted. *Second* are "behavior constraints." Each culture has its own rules about appropriate behavior which affect verbal and nonverbal communication. Whether one looks the opposite person within the eye or not; whether one says what one means overtly or talks round the issue; and the way close the people stand to every other once they are talking are practices that differ from culture to culture. *Third* being "emotional constraints." Different cultures regulate the display of emotion differently. Members of some cultures get very emotional after they are debating a problem. They yell, exhibit their anger, fear, frustration, etc openly. Other cultures try and keep their emotions hidden, exhibiting or sharing only the "rational" or factual aspects of matters.

Steps in Health Communication Process

The health communication process will be complicated, but like all complex process the health communication effort will be counteracted into variety of discrete steps. By developing an understanding of those steps the method can become infinitely more manageable. The sections below outline the assorted steps involved—from getting down to end—in the method. While they're presented in fairly strict sequence, it should be realized that there are situations during which the sequence can be changed or, in rare circumstances, a step be eliminated.

Stages within the Health Communication Process

The health communication process will be divided into several distinct stages. For our purposes, we are able to consider these stages as: planning, development, implementation, and evaluation.

(a) Stage of planning

A carefully devised plan will enable the project to provide meaningful results. Taking the time to carefully plan the project will ultimately save time by defining program objectives and indicating steps for meeting those objectives. whether or not the project is an element of a broader health promotion effort, a concept specific to the communication component is important. Indeed, any health communication effort should fit within the context of the organization's overall marketing plan and be told by its strategic plan.

Stating the matter

Defining the matter or the problem is that the critical opening within the plan development process. It involves identifying the "real" issues at hand and therefore the specific information required for the event of the communication initiative. Unless the problem is correctly defined, the probabilities of developing a successful campaign are low. Time spent initially isolating the problems represents a decent investment

Stating Assumptions:

One among the critical steps at the outset is that the stating of assumptions. "Assumptions" are the understandings that drive the design process, and, if they're not specified early within the process, the communication team may find itself well down the road holding conflicting notions of what the project is absolutely about. Assumptions can relate to demographic trends, reimbursement practices, and any number of other aspects of the healthcare system. Assumptions also should be made about the audience that's being targeted. These would come with assumptions associated with the character of the population, the political climate, other options for services. Some assumptions can–and should–be stated at the outset of the design process. Others are going to be developed as information is collected and more in-depth knowledge is gained concerning the community, its healthcare needs, and its resources. Although assumptions will undoubtedly be refined because the planning process continues, it's important to start with a minimum of general assumptions identified.

Reviewing Available Data

Gaps in available information should be noted and sources of additional information identified. the categories of sources of data are going to be determined by the kind of issue being addressed within the communication project. The kinds of data that ought to be compiled at this stage include:

The incidence or prevalence of the ill health.
The characteristics of these laid low with the identified problem
The implications of the pathological state for people, communities and even the healthcare system
The possible causes for the condition.

The possible solutions, treatments, or interventions. Both published and unpublished reports is also available from internal and external sources. variety of federal health information clearinghouses and Websites provide information, products, materials, and sources of further assistance for specific health subjects. A helpful start in assessing the matter could also be to access the suitable websites and relevant health agencies to get information on the health issue being addressed. It is seldom necessary to *"reinventing the wheel"* in a world where there's virtually nothing new under the sun. Therefore, it's useful to spot other organizations that are addressing the identical issue and determine the categories of communication initiatives they need underway.

Objectives of Communication

Once communication objectives are defined and circulated, they function a form of contract or agreement about the aim of the communication and establish the categories of outcomes to be measured. Objectives ask the precise targets to be reached in support of goal attainment. While goals are general statements, objectives have to be very specific and stated in clear and concise terms. Objectives must even be time bound, with clear deadlines established for his or her accomplishment. They have to be amenable to evaluation. within the case of communication initiatives, the objectives should be reasonable and reachable and clearly associated with the change desired.

Evaluating the Health Communication Approach

In some cases, health communication alone may accomplish little or nothing without policy, technological, or infrastructure changes. In some instances, effective solutions might not yet exist for a communication program to support. for instance, no treatment may exist for an illness, or an answer may require services that aren't yet available. In these cases, the health communication program should be redirected to support the significance of research issues of relevance. Raising awareness or increasing knowledge among individuals or the organizations that serve them is usually easily accomplished through the communication process. However, accomplishing such an objective might not necessarily result in behavior change. as an example, it's unreasonable to expect communication to cause a sustained change in complex behaviors or catch up on a scarcity of health services, products, or resources. The power and willingness of the intended audience to form certain changes also affect the reasonableness of assorted communication objectives.

Determining the Intended listeners

The effort to find out the intended audience will determine who is most affected, who is at the high risk, and what other factors contribute to the matter. Intended populations are usually defined vividly, using just some descriptors (e.g., women over age 50). Intended audiences are often carved out of those broad population groups and defined more narrowly supported characteristics like attitudes, demographics, geographical area, or patterns of behavior. Examples might include physically inactive adolescents, heavy smokers with low education and income levels who are fatalistic about health issues, or urban African-American men with hypertension who board the South. Because the intended audience's ability and willingness to create a behavior change affects the extent to which communication objectives are reasonable and realistic, it's most effective to pick out intended audiences and develop communication objectives in tandem.

Deducing a method

At some point during this process, the selection strategy must be considered. The strategy refers to the generalized approach to communication that's to be taken in response to the challenges identified. This could mean choosing between a public health strategy, a free market approach, an academic model, or a public/private consortium approach. The strategy should provide overall direction for the initiative, fit the available resources, minimize resistance, reach the acceptable targeted groups, and, ultimately, accomplish the goals of the communication initiative. While the precise strategic approach to be taken might not be specified at this time, a minimum of the choices are often narrowed. this may serve to focus subsequent planning activities by eliminating strategies that are considered unproductive. as an example, it's going to are determined that the target population must be educated on the problems before attempting behavioral change. A communication strategy should include everything one must know to speak with the intended audience. It defines the intended audience, identifies the actions its members should take, tells how they're going to benefit (from their perspective, not necessarily from a public health perspective), and the way they'll most effectively be reached. Developing the strategy statement provides a decent test of whether the project has enough information to start developing messages. It also gives the communication team a chance to get management and partner buy-in for the approach. Having an approved strategy statement will save time and energy later.

Selecting the correct sort of Appeal

There are a range of how within which to capture the intended audience's attention. Appeals may be made to their emotions, their intellect, or their pocketbooks. The most effective approach depends on the character of the intended audience's preferences, the kind of data being communicated and, ultimately, what the project hopes to accomplish. Positive emotional appeals show the advantages of communicating right things to intended audience members who will gain after they take the action portrayed within the message. Research has shown that, in general, messages that present a significant benefit but don't address any drawbacks tend to be most appropriate when intended audience members are already in favor of a plan or practice. Humorous appeals can work for easy messages, especially if most competing communication isn't humorous. The humor should be appropriate for the health issue and convey the correct message; otherwise, people tend to recollect the joke but not the message. Threat (or fear) appeals are shown to be effective with two groups. Such appeals tend to be more practical with "copers" (people who aren't anxious by nature) and "sensation seekers" (certain youth), and when exposure to the message is voluntary (e.g., discovering a brochure instead of mandatory attendance at a drug abuse prevention program).

(b) Stage of Development

The development stage has its own important aspects of project development

Materials Development

Developing and pretesting messages and materials are important because they indicate early within the process which messages are going to be simplest with the intended audiences. Knowing this may save time and money. Positive results from pretesting may also generate early buy-in from others within the organization. it's beneficial to start out with existing materials, if possible, and determine what could also be appropriate for the actual project instead of reinventing the wheel. Considering the magnitude of this task, existing communication logistics (booklets, leaflets, posters, public service announcements, videotapes) should be inventoried. It should be possible to search out existing materials available from health departments, voluntary health organizations, health care provider associations, and other sources. Using the communication strategy statement as a guide, the subsequent questions could also be posed with relevancy any existing materials:

Are the messages accurate, current, complete, and relevant?
Are the materials appropriate for the intended audience in terms of format, style, cultural considerations, and readability level?
Are the materials likely to satisfy the communication objectives?

Once concepts regarding message are established for the intended audience, the material formats (e.g., brochure, videotape) which will best suit the project should be ascertained. These materials should be evaluated in terms of:

The character of the message (e.g., its complexity, sensitivity, style)
The function of the message (e.g., to show to a difficulty or to teach a brand new skill)
The activities and channels previously selected
The budget and other available resources
The development of latest materials typically represents a significant expenditure.

Formats should be chosen that the program can afford. it's important to avoid overspending on materials production so as to afford sufficient quantities, distribution expenses, and process evaluation. Knowledge of the intended audience should be accustomed combine, adapt, and devise new ways to urge the message across. Input should be sought from the intended audience or partners with relation to decisions about materials.

Planning and Launch:

It's important to plan for distribution, promotion, and process evaluation. The character of the project might get pleasure from a quiet, low-key launch, or its nature may mandate a significant kick-off event. A kickoff event can help to create broader awareness regarding the program and promote community involvement. Kickoff events are a wonderful thanks to develop relationships with those who could also be willing to induce involved within the program. Scheduling an occasion also creates a deadline, which is able to help the program avoid unnecessary lag time or protracted preparations. In order to boost media coverage for a kickoff event, variety of steps may be taken. for instance, the organization might create a news "hook" or angle that creates the event newsworthy, inform the media of the event during a timely manner, create media kits to facilitate accurate reporting of the difficulty, and include the total range of appropriate media. These would come with precise media portals, like Newspapers, TV stations, radio, health-related publications (the trade press), foreign language publications or broadcast media, Internet, and websites, and organization publications.

(c) Stage of implementation

The payoff of planning comes within the implementation of the plan. The planning process creates a road map which the communication staff uses to maneuver the initiative to where it must be. it's during the implementation stage, however, that the method often breaks down. The oft-repeated maxim that "the last plan continues to be sitting on the shelf" generally reflects poor implementation instead of any flaw within the plan itself. The transition from aiming to implementation involves a hand-off from the design team to the management team. Implementation must occur at different levels and at different sectors of the divisions of the organization. For this reason, the implementation of the plan requires tier of coordination that few organizations have in situ. An implementation matrix may be developed employing a spreadsheet and may lay out who is to try and do what and once they are to do it. The matrix should list every action entailed by the plan, breaking each action down into tasks, if appropriate. For each action or task the responsible party should be identified, together with any secondary parties that ought to be involved during this activity. The matrix should indicate resource requirements (in terms of staff time, money and other resources). the beginning and end dates for this activity should be identified. Any prerequisites for accomplishing this task should be identified at the outset and factored into the project plan. Finally, benchmarks should be established that allow the design team to see when the activity has been completed. The nature of the progress indicators used are going to be determined by the kind of plan.

The plan developed to manage the campaign should indicate how and when resources are going to be needed, when specific events will occur, and at what points you'll assess your efforts. On-going process evaluation will determine the extent to which activities are being completed at scheduled times, the intended audiences are being reached, which activities or materials are most successful, and which aspects of the program must be altered or eliminated.

Message delivery channels have changed significantly in recent years (National Cancer Institute, 2003). Today, channels are more numerous, are often more narrowly focused on an intended audience, and represent changes that have occurred in supplying, the mass media, and society. Interpersonal channels (e.g., physicians, friends, family members, clergy, and coaches of the intended audiences) put health messages in a simple and familiar context. These channels are more likely to be trusted and influential than media sources.

(d) Stage of Evaluation

Evaluating the communication project should be top of mind on the primary day of operating, and therefore the means for evaluation should be built into the method itself. Evaluation is important to see the efficiency of the method and therefore the effectiveness of the initiative.

Evaluation techniques focus to 2 kinds of analysis: process (or formative) analysis and outcome (or summative) analysis. The former evaluates systems, procedures, communication processes, and other factors that contribute to the efficient operation of a program. Outcome evaluation focuses more on end results or what's ultimately accomplished. Process evaluation essentially measures efficiency, while outcome evaluation measures effectiveness (Adams and Schvaneveldt, 1991).

Evaluation should involve on-going monitoring of the communication process, including benchmarks and/or milestones for assessment along the way. this may require the clarification of the objectives and goals of the initiative.

Data collection and benchmarking are extremely important for measuring progress in meeting objectives, and documenting the method of change is an ongoing task that ought to occur on a daily basis.

Health communicators should submit updates to the key parties involved within the initiative. Once the inquiries to be answered through the evaluation are identified, the following step is to choose which methods will best address those questions. a number of the methods to be utilized include: monitoring and feedback system; surveys about the initiative; report on attainment of goals; surveys on behavior; interviews with key participants; and community-level indicators of impact. Although evaluation techniques are often praised for his or her bottom-line objectivity, they're also useful in healthcare where it's out of the question to position a dollar value on everything. Thus, cost-effectiveness analysis can relate the intangible aspects of the communication initiative in its evaluation. Thus, strict cost/benefit analyses are likely to be less relevant to be used in healthcare as compared to other industries.

References

Adams, G. R. and Schvaneveldt. J. D. (1991). *Understanding research methods*. New York: Congman.
National Cancer Institute. (2003). *Making health communication work*. Washington: US Government Printing Office.
University of Kansas. (N.D.) Community tool box. Web-based planning guide.
URL: http://ctb.lsi.ukans.edu.
Berkowitz, Eric. (1996). Essentials of health care marketing. Gaithersburg, MD: Aspen.
Daniel O'Keefe. (1990). Persuasion: Theory and research. Newbury Park, CA: Sage.
Ting-Toomey, Stella. (Ed.) (1994). Challenge of facework: Cross-cultural and interpersonal issues.
Albany, NY: State University of recent York Press.
Berkowitz, Eric N. 1996. Essentials of health care marketing. Gaithersburg, MD: Aspen Publishers.
Berkowitz, Eric N., and Hillestad, Steven G. (1991). Healthcare marketing plans: From strategy to action. Boston: Jones and Bartlett.
Eisenberg, D., and R. C. Kessler (1993). Unconventional medicine within the us. New England Journal of drugs, 328, 246–252.
Fishbein, M., & Ajzen, I. (1975). Belief, attitude, intention and behavior: An introduction to theory and research. Reading, MA: Addison-Wesley.
Maslow, Abraham 1970. Motivation and personality (2nd ed.). New York: Harper & Row.
National Cancer Institute. (2003). Making health communication work. Washington, DC: US Government Printing Office.
National Center for Health Statistics. (2002). Health u. s., 2002. Washington, DC: US Government Printing Office.
McKinley, John, & Sonja J. McKinley. (1977). The questionable contribution of medical measures to the decline of mortality in the united states in the twentieth century. *Milbank Memorial Fund Quarterly/ Health and Society*, 405–428.
Thomas, Richard K. (2004). *Marketing health services*. Chicago: Health Administration Press

CHAPTER 4

Transactional Analysis and Conflict Management

Dr Nilanjana Ghosh

Assistant Professor, Dept of Community and Family Medicine,

All India Institute of Medical Sciences, Guwahati

INTRODUCTION

Communication is the backbone of human existence. Management skills deal with the art of effective communication. It has been noted that many discrepancies arise and also get solved by appropriate use of verbal and nonverbal communication skills. However, the basis behind the crossed interactions are very scientific and has been zeroed down to the fact that every person has three types of ego in them (P, C, and A viz. parent ego, child ego, and adult ego). Interactions with other people — when they happen on the same platforms — seldom cause conflict, but transactions that occur between the parent ego of one person and the child ego of another can certainly lead to conflict. Hence, in order to understand and resolve interpersonal conflicts in hospitals, basic concepts of transaction need to be analysed well.

Rebellious or timid behaviour occur when parent ego clashes with child ego of another. Interpersonal conflicts occur more in the case of Crossed Transactions.

Here are certain examples:

  - X: I need to go to market just now (Child ego)
  - Y: No, you can't, it's raining severely (Parent ego)
  - X: Who are you to stop me, I am going (Child ego)
  - Y: Do whatever you want to then, don't ask me (Parent ego)

Interpersonal conflicts are far less in the case of complimentary transactions, as mature interactions occur when egos of the same plane from both participants interact.

Here are certain examples:

  - X: Please close the door, I am going to the market (Adult ego)
  - Y: Are you sure, it's raining severely (Adult ego)

X: Oh, thank you, but I will be carrying an umbrella (Adult ego)

Y: Ok, don't get wet, take care, and let me know if I can be of any help (Adult ego)

In the afore-mentioned context, it becomes clear that not only communication but a deep insight into the type of interactions leads to a clear picture of the working dynamics of an organisation. The leader needs to be empathetic, emotionally intelligent and sensitive to the needs of the employers to ensure a healthy working environment[1-2].

Yet, conflicts ensue in almost every set up and hence, conflict management becomes mandatory to resolve them and attain targets in stipulated deadlines through concerted teamwork.

Conflict Management[3-6]

Hospitals have huge potentials of conflicts given the varied manpower, job diversification, range of logistics and the huge infrastructure running 24*7 without any break. Researchers have proven that hospital administrators have devoted 20 per cent of their time to resolving conflicts. Sources may range from discrete to perceptions, and these are usually an indication of some unresolved issues which need to be addressed. This dysfunctional and unproductive issue needs to be nipped at the bud before it can loom large and threaten goal attainment and affect the outcomes.

Conflicts can occur at any level because of disagreement over what goals need to be attained, what roles need to be performed and what methods to be accomplish in a hospital. The process of conflict is hence attempted to be put into five stages:

Stage 1: *Potential Opposition* — antecedent conditions being communication, structure (leadership style, goals), personal variables (attitude, make up, value systems)

Stage 2: *Cognition and Personalisation* — perceived and felt conflict

Stage 3: *Intentions of Conflict Handling*—competing, collaborating, compromising, avoiding, accommodating

Stage 4: *Behaviour* — overt conflict depending on own/other's behaviour

Stage 5: *Outcome* — functional outcome/dysfunctional outcome

Hence, the next major issue that one needs to tackle is how to handle said conflicts; this can best be done through the five types of Conflict Handling Orientations as suggested by K Thomas when put on coordinates of Cooperativeness on X axis from low to high (moving left to right) and Assertiveness on Y axis from low to high (moving from bottom to top):

(a) Competition (Win – Lose)

(b) Avoidance (Lose – Lose)

(c) Compromise

(d) Collaboration (Win –Win)

(e) Accommodation (Lose –Win)

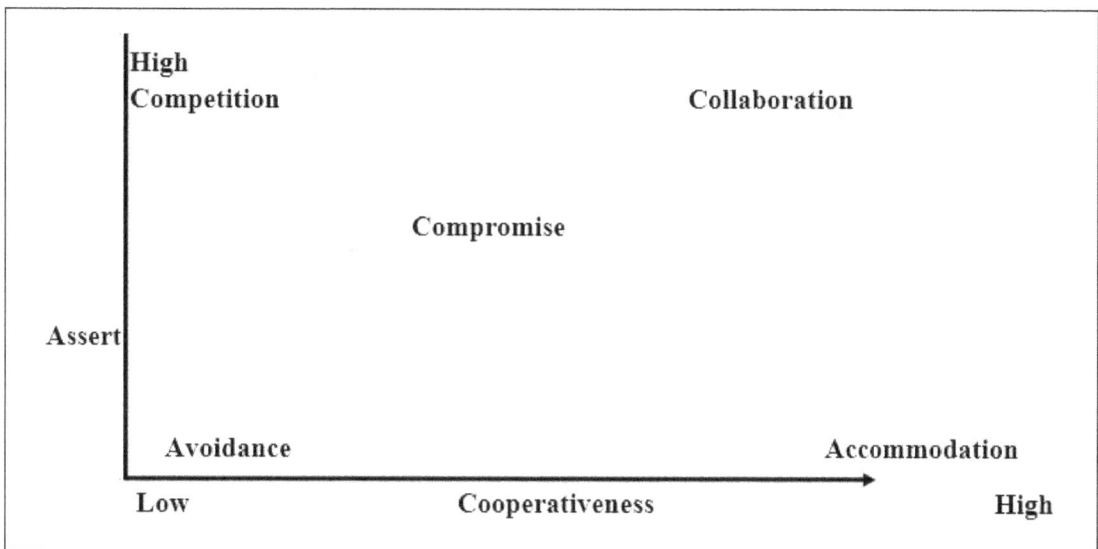

Hence, as different types of handling techniques exist depending on the different types of leaders, the outcomes vary significantly. Even types of conflicts can be categorised broadly into a few subtypes, namely:

Intrapersonal Conflict: This depends on the frustration levels and hence the defense mechanisms like aggression, withdrawal, fixation, compromise and displacements (redirecting pent up emotions) exist. It can be resolved by insightful counselling.

Role Conflict: It has been seen that 62 per cent of all conflicts arise from here due to nondescript or compartmentalised professional roles, personal roles, team/work-group roles. Hence, clarifying their perceptions and expectations, renegotiating role assignments with related skills and examining overlapping roles are the key to combat it.

Goal Conflict: This usually occurs when the team of clinicians decide a quality of care and it comes in way with the organisational goal set by the institution. Hence, timely meetings and clear discussions frequently are needed to monitor the situation and formulate common goals. It can be resolved by management by objective and role definitions.

Inter Group Conflict: Hospitals have heterogeneity of personnel, interdependence, authority level, perception of service units, all different from one another, which may lead to such conflicts. It can be resolved by participative management team and training sensitivity programme.

Client Hospital Conflict: Inability of public health care delivery to provide for all quality care at suboptimal range and contradictions among patients as beneficiary/consumers is the main reason of such conflict. This can be resolved by community goal setting, public relations and OPD programme.

Interpersonal Conflict[5]: Conflicts stem from human emotions to offsetting efforts mainly due to perception difference or gaps in communication. These majorly include interpersonal disagreement and interpersonal antagonism.

It can be resolved by

- Transactional Analysis, which goes a long way in resolving it
- Creative problem solving, aka, assertive behaviour training
- Johari Window Model, which is a model by Luft and Igham that analyses interactions between self and others and goes a long way in conflict resolution

Known to Self Known to Others **OPEN SELF**	Known to Self Unknown to Others **HIDDEN SELF**
Unknown to Self Known to Others **BLIND SELF**	Unknown to Self Unknown to Others **Undiscovered**

Organisational Conflict: This deals with hospital per se

- *Status-related Conflict* – particularly with women, minorities and specialists and basic doctors
- *Functional Conflict* – between functional departments in hospital
- *Hierarchical Conflict* – lateral dimension hierarchies being undefined creates conflicts
- *Competing Goals* – when employee has two or more needs confronting each other like approach conflict, approach avoid conflict and avoid conflict

Hence conflict was, is and will be. Authentic communication and respect for difference of opinion is required for smooth functioning of an organisation to attain the formulated goals.

References

1. Janet Moursund. *The Process of Counseling and Therapy*. New Jersey: Prentice – Hall, Inc Eaglewood Cliffs, 1985.

2. S Robbins. *Managing Organizational Conflict*. New Jersey: Eaglewood Cliffs: Prentice Hall,1974.

3. RJ Burke. 'Methods of Resolving Superior Subordinate Conflict: The Constructive Use of Subordinate Differences and Disagreements'. *Organizational Behaviour and Human Performance 5*, pp 393-411. 1970.

4. DH Nath, R Bagga, AG Chandorkar and N Dhar. *Introduction to Management and Human Resource Development: Theme I, Block 3*. National Institute of Health and Family Welfare, Distance Learning: Certificate Course in Hospital Management, 2009.

5. SP Robbins. *Organizational Behaviour, Concept, Controversies and Applications* (5th ed). New Delhi: Practice Hall of India, Pvt. Ltd,1991.

CHAPTER 5

Inventory Management

Dr B Venkatashiva Reddy

Assistant Professor, Department of Community and Family Medicine

All India Institute of Medical Sciences Mangalagiri, Andhra Pradesh

INTRODUCTION

An inventory is a detailed, itemised list of assets held by a hospital. Inventory management is an approach designed to keep track of inventory movement. Through the concept of inventory management, one can understand a hospital's use for products such as medications, supplies, dressing material, disposables and general stores in the hospital. Inventory management is required to take care of the cost and vitality of the drugs in the hospital. It means storing a sufficient number of products needed by different units, such as medications or supplies.

The purpose of hospital inventory management is to ensure the supply of products at the optimum cost anywhere in the hospital at any time. Prices should be optimised in order to provide appropriate product costs to minimise dead stock and obsolescence by analysing retaining costs, purchasing costs and stocking costs. The whole concept is the availability of goods that hold prices to a minimum.

Inventory Cost

Purchase Cost: It is the real cost of materials such as medicines, linen or every other store. The aim is to minimise this price without losing efficiency, which can be achieved by buying in bulk, by generic name and by government vendors and portals.

Carrying Cost: Stock carrying costs will be the expense of interest on capital spent on material, transportation costs, insurance costs, labour costs to manage inventory, obsolescence such as expiry medications, etc. To minimise healthcare expenses, the carrying costs should be low.

Ordering Cost: There is money spent on procurement, such as workers participating, stationery expenses, computing time, etc. The ordering expense does not depend on the quantity of the merchandise.

Stock Out Cost: In the case of stock out, cost of higher prices and additional work made for the goods procured during the emergency.

Objective of Inventory Management

The objectives of inventory management are dead stock or perishability prevention for an acceptable level of inventory, storage cost optimisation, thereby decreasing the odds of retaining unnecessary stock, maintaining enough stock, enhancement of cash flow, and reducing the cost value of inventories via discounts and other advantages to reduce price.

Types of Inventory Management

Bar-code Inventory Management	Continuous Inventory Management	Periodic Inventory Management
Automated and simplified version using software	To track the direction of material movement, it links the barcode and radio frequency identification with the accounting inventory system, inventory received, and point of sales systems together with the manufacturing system	Manual process to determine the closing inventory value in the financial year

Techniques of Inventory Management

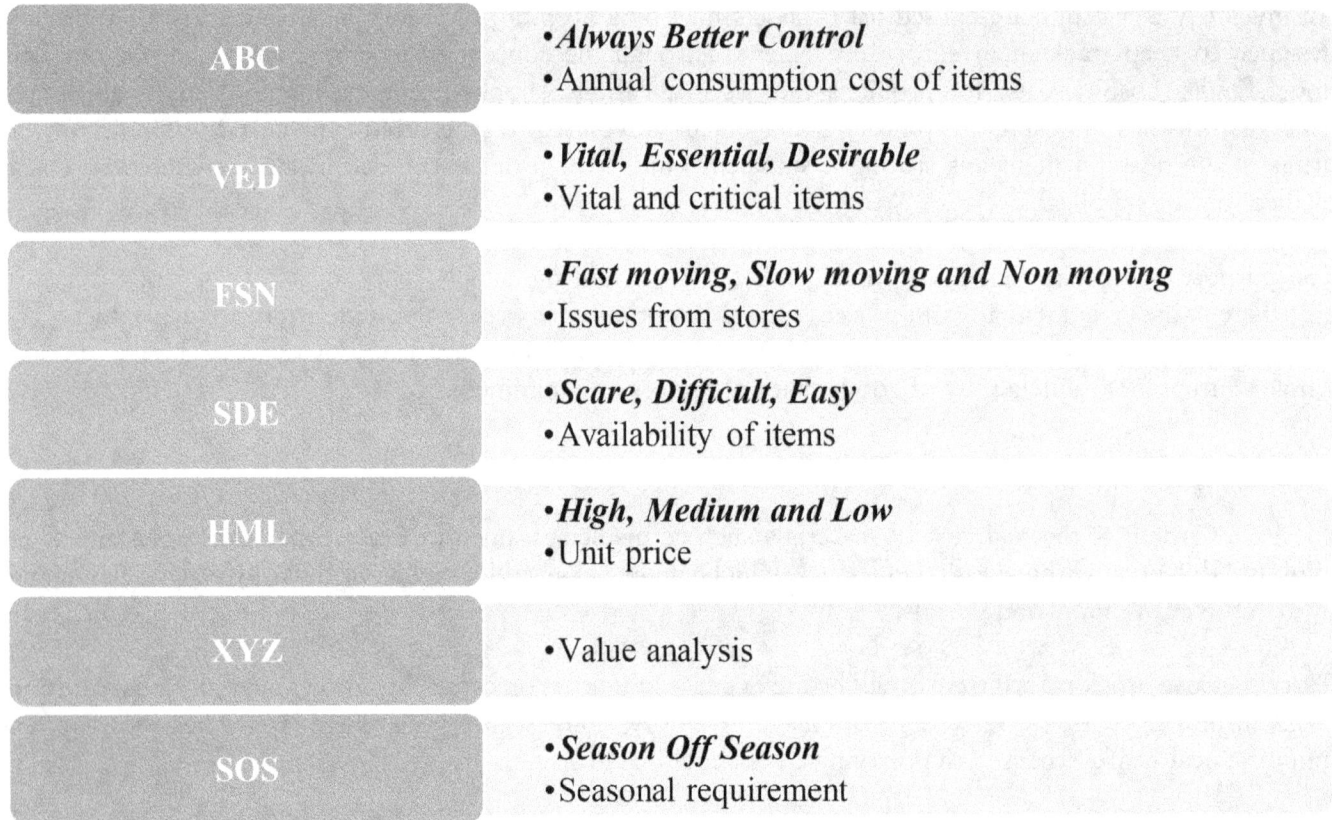

ABC
- *Always Better Control*
- Annual consumption cost of items

VED
- *Vital, Essential, Desirable*
- Vital and critical items

FSN
- *Fast moving, Slow moving and Non moving*
- Issues from stores

SDE
- *Scare, Difficult, Easy*
- Availability of items

HML
- *High, Medium and Low*
- Unit price

XYZ
- Value analysis

SOS
- *Season Off Season*
- Seasonal requirement

Factors Determining Inventory Management

Factors influencing the management of inventory are degree of specialisation and distinction at various stages of the commodity, capability and versatility of systems, capacity of output and facility of storage, the essence of the method of production, amount of scarcity defense, organisation factors, characteristics of the fabrication method and additional considerations.

Functions of Inventory Management

The major functional facets of inventory control include prioritisation of ABC items, accounting and tax activities related to central store management, installation and control of barcodes, supervision of inventory handling, preservation of information on serial numbers of goods, management of inventory lists, real-life real-time central store records, real-time location tracking of goods, replenishment process, specification of products, their ID numbers and forms and synchronisation with central store stock.

ABC (Always Better Control) Technique

The theory of Pareto states that a small quantity of goods typically implies a significant amount of expense and vice versa.

When we treat our supplies at our pharmacy, such as drugs, the total annual cost of the various medicines is also categorised.

(a) 10 per cent of the medications would cost 70 per cent of the overall currency (Group A commodities).

(b) 20 per cent of the medications would cost about 20 per cent of the overall currency (Group B commodities).

(c) 70 per cent of medications will cost only 10 per cent of the overall currency (Group C commodities).

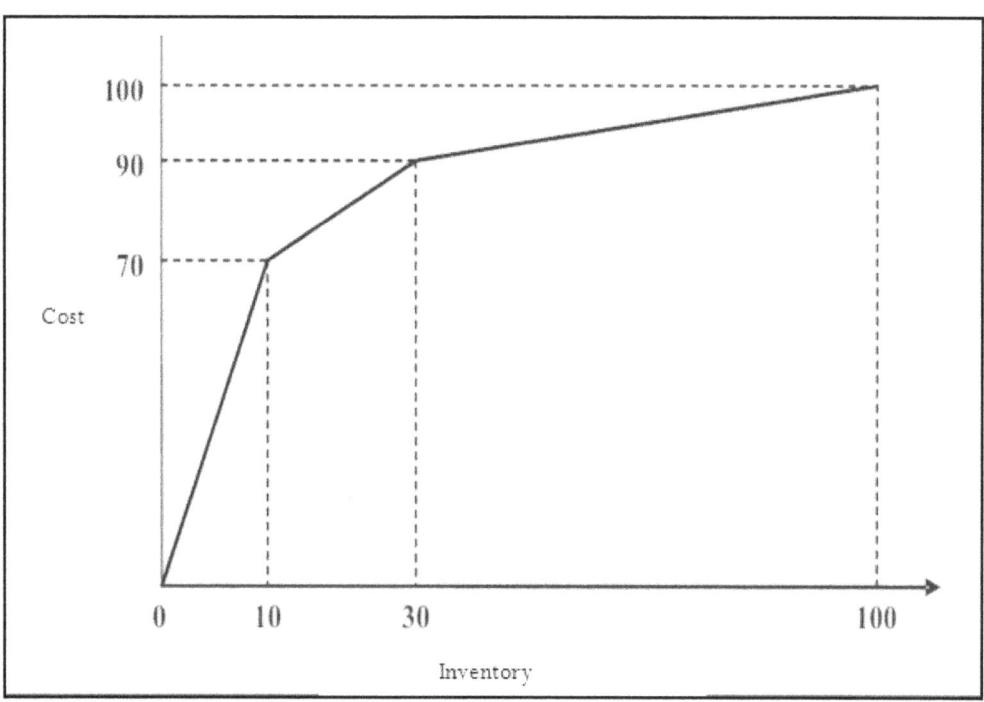

The first is the estimation of the annual expense of each drug.

The pharmaceutical goods are then organised at the negative value of the annual gross expense. That implies that the top will be the most expensive and the bottom will be the least expensive.

Then the total cost is estimated and a table is drawn up (Table 1).

It can be shown from Table - 1 above that about 10 per cent of drugs will cost 70 per cent of the overall annual cost. These are considered the goods of Category A. The remaining 20 per cent of goods would cost nearly 20 per cent of the annual net cost. These are called goods of Category B. Just 10 per cent of the gross annual expenditure is paid for by the remaining 70 per cent of goods. These are the C commodities group.

S NO	PRODUCT	COST INR	% COST	CATEGORY
1.	Inj Taxim	9,000	19.5	
2.	Tab Azithromycin	8,500	18.4	
3.	Inj Monocef	8,300	18.0	
4.	Inj Insulin	8,000	17.3	
5.	InjAlteplase	5,000	10.8	A
6.	Oint soframycin	7,000	15.2	B
7.	Bandage Cotton	400	0.9	C
	Total	46,200		

VED Analysis (Vital, Essential, And Desirable)

A medication with low cost and low use is observed in hospitals, but it is nevertheless lifesaving. As per the ABC study, we should not disregard those drugs just because they fall under the category of community C. For instance, in a month, Anti Rabies Immunoglobulin can be used very rarely. It has an annual cost that is very modest, but it is critical and life-saving. It should be available round the clock in any hospital. ABC-VED analysis was done for this purpose.

	V items	E items	D items	
A Items	AV	AE	AD	Category 1 Items
B Items	BV	BE	BD	Category 2 Items
C Items	CV	CE	CD	Category 3 Items

Economic Order Quantity (EOQ)

In order to reduce product costs such as keeping costs, scarcity costs, and order costs, economic order quantity (EOQ) is the optimal order quantity that a hospital can buy. The formula for EOQ is:

Where:

Q = EOQ units
D = Demand in units (typically on an annual basis)
S = Order cost (per purchase order)
H = Holding costs (per unit, per year)

$$Q = \sqrt{\frac{2SD}{H}}$$

The timing of reordering, the cost of making an order and the cost of storage is taken into account by EOQ. If a hospital places small orders to retain a certain volume of inventory, the cost of buying is greater, and more store space is required. For e.g., consider that a hospital vaccinates patients and that community requiring 1,000 vials each year. Holding a vial of vaccine in storage costs the hospital INR 50 a year, and the fixed cost for placing an order is INR 20. The EOQ formula is the square root of (2 x 1,000 vial x INR 20 order cost)/ (INR 50 holding cost) or 28.3 with rounding. The ideal order size to minimise costs and meet demand is slightly more than 28 vials of vaccine.

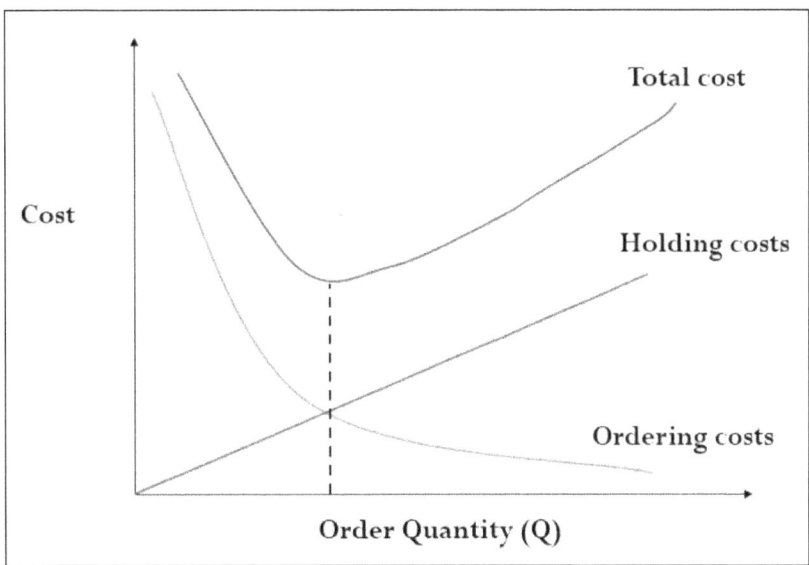

Reorder Time

While the quantity formula of the economic order points to the cost-effective sum of stock required, the reorder time formula determines the correct time to order the products. There's a formula here:

Lead time demand + Safety stock = Reorder time

Lead Time

The lead time is a number of days after you have placed an order with your supplier for the stock order to be shipped to your central store. This indicator is important for hospitals. It becomes critical during any breakdowns in infrastructure, strikes, market spikes or seasonal deliveries. Multiply two figures to measure the lead time demand: the lead time for a given commodity and the estimated daily consumption of this item.

Safety Stock

This is a cushion, or a buffer of supplies available in hospital, and is called security storage. Multiply the highest (maximum) daily intake of an item and the highest lead time for this item to measure this (in days). Then, multiply an item's daily total intake and average lead time (in days). Finally, from the first figure, deduct the latter. This discrepancy — in items/units — is your protection stock number.

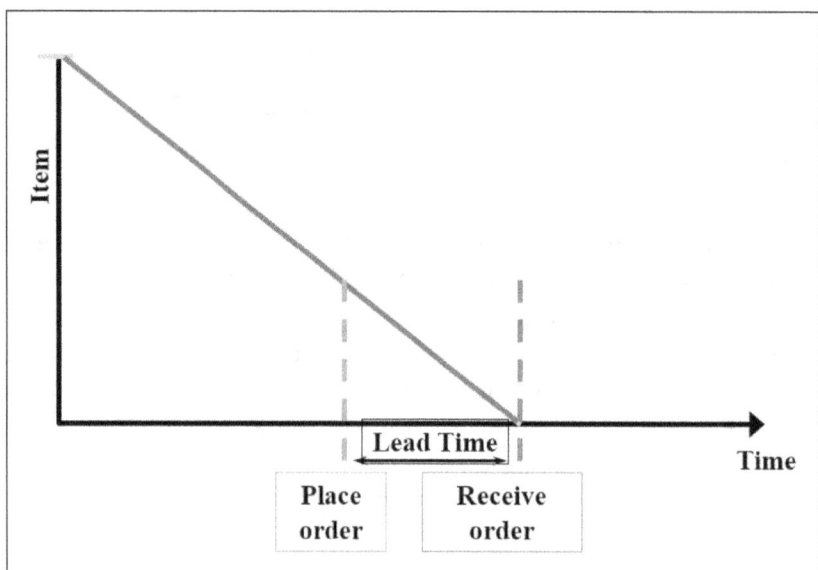

Here's an example. You sell the COVID 19 vaccine at your pharmacy in Andhra Pradesh. The dealer works in Delhi. It normally takes 30 days to ship the products to Andhra Pradesh from Delhi (average lead time). Often it takes 50 days to ship the items during holidays, or market spikes, or strikes or something (highest lead time).

On average, you sell five COVID 19 vaccine vials per day (the average daily intake) and the peak amount of sales you have during holiday times is 10 COVID 19 vaccines per day (highest daily consumption). So, the formula of your safety stock looks like this:

10x50 - 5x30 = 500-150 = 350 5x30 (units)

Government e-Market (GeM)

DGS&D has developed the GeM portal for the procurement of both goods and services with the technological assistance of the National e-Governance Division (Ministry of Electronics and Information Technology). The platform was unveiled by the Minister of Commerce and Industry on 9th August 2016. More than 7400 goods in nearly 150 product groups and transport sector procurement options are currently available on the GeM POC platform. GeM is a fully paperless, cashless and system-driven e-market position that allows for limited human interface procurement of general use products and services.

E-Aushadhi

E-Aushadhi is a full web-based supply chain management solution for medication, surgical and suture delivery to various District Drug Warehouses (DWH), medical schools, hospitals, Community Health Centers (CHC), Primary Health Centers (PHC) and Drug Distribution Centers (DDC) from which the drugs are delivered to patients.

References

1. https://afifnurichwan.files.wordpress.com/2015/06/inventory-control-and-management-second-edition.pdf
2. DV Devine, GD Sher, HW Reesink, S Panzer, PA Hetzel, JK Wong, M Horvath, et.al. *Inventory Management*. Vox Sang. 2010 Apr; 98 (3 Pt 1):e295-363.
3. R Levin. *Inventory Control,* Sep;135 (9): 1319-20. J Am Dent Assoc, 2004.
4. https://www.india.gov.in/spotlight/government-e-marketplace-procurement-made-smart#tab=tab-1
5. https://apps.nic.in/apps/government/eaushadhi

CHAPTER 6

Time and Stress Management

Dr. Parmeshwar Satpathy

Assistant Professor, Department of Community Medicine

Dr. B.C. Roy Multi-Speciality Medical Research Centre, IIT Kharagpur, West Bengal

INTRODUCTION

In today's fast paced world full of newer technological advances and challenges on a daily basis, we often come across health care professionals complaining about being overburdened by work due to lack of time ultimately resulting in stress and decreased productivity. Medical education curriculum in India does not inculcate time-management skills amongst medical undergraduates and postgraduates. The focus remains on acquiring knowledge and new skills so much so that an important aspect of time management is rarely a consideration.

As the healthcare system continues to change, healthcare professionals are overburdened with an increasing number of administrative and management responsibilities. Time management and stress are closely intertwined. Effective time management goes a long way in reducing stress and increasing the overall productivity and vice-versa.(1,2)1987 (Fig 1)

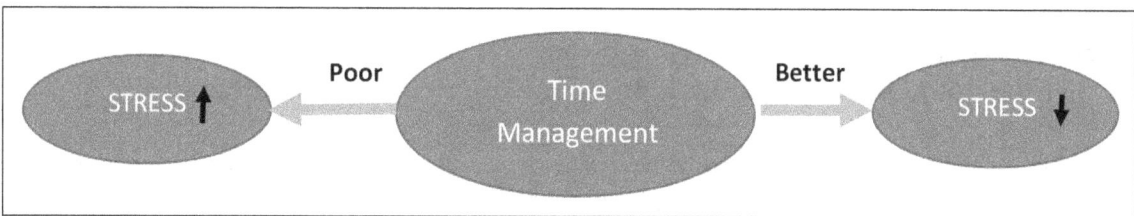

Fig.1: Relationship between time management and Stress

Time management is an art and health care professionals should master this art in order to lead a stress free and productive life. There is always a lot of scope for better management of available time. Time management is the process of organizing our lives so that we devote more time on activities that are really important to us; and minimize the time we spend on things of minimal importance. It is basically doing smart work in the available time.

Effective time management eventually leads to decreased stress, increased recreation, more contentment and greater success. Every professional gets the same amount of time each day. Every work that an individual does, requires time, and the more successful people use their time intelligently. With growing emphasis on efficiency and effectiveness in health care, how a health care professional manages his/her time is an important consideration.(3)

The 4ds of Effectiveness

For time management methods to prove successful one needs to have the 4Ds of Effectiveness.(4) (Fig 2)

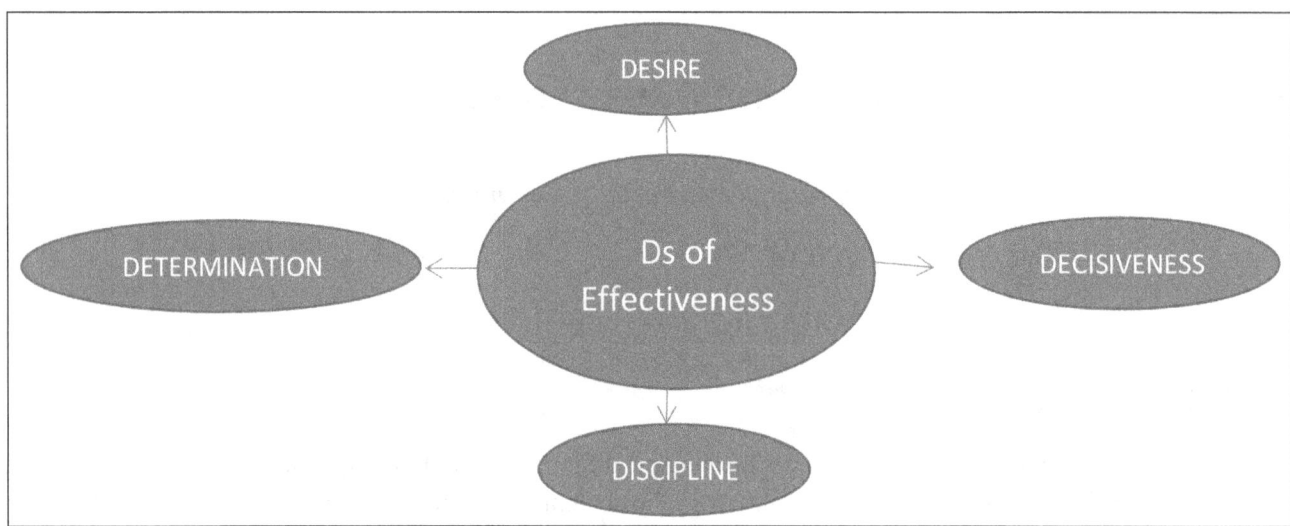

Fig 2. 4Ds of Effectiveness

- Desire: An individual must have a passionate desire to get time under control.
- Decisiveness: An individual must make a clear decision to rehearse good time management techniques.
- Determination: There should be a strong determination to excel in time management techniques.
- Discipline: One must discipline himself/herself to make time management a routine and lifelong practice.

Significance of Time Management

Time management is fundamental for wellbeing of an individual. How much one feels in charge of his/her time and life is a significant determinant of his/her degree of inward harmony, happiness and mental peace.

By learning how to manage his/her time one will be able to lead a more balanced life, have more leisure time, meet deadlines, overcome procrastination, reduce stress and accomplish significant life and career goals. Learning and practicing time-management techniques will have huge benefits throughout an individual's career.

Time Management Strategies

Good time management is fundamental for coping with the pressures of modern day life without encountering undue stress. Time management strategies are basically based on two principles, Pareto's Principle and Parkinson's Law. Pareto's principle was given by Italian economist Vilfredo Pareto. According to this principle or the 80/20 rule, 20% of energy brings about 80% of desired results.(5,6) This clarifies the fact that we accomplish the majority of our goals with a minimal amount of energy. According to Parkinson's Law, human beings have a natural tendency to expend more effort on trivial things that are perceived as necessary rather than those that are truly important.(7) Proper time management does not mean accomplishing more work. It implies to focus on the tasks that are really very important. In one's job as well as in life as a whole, determining how to manage time effectively will help an individual feel less stressful and more relaxed and focused.

Following are the various strategies for better time management:(4,6)

- **Study how time is spent:** Time spent on various activities during any working day can be assessed by carrying out time-utilization studies. For a health manager, this activity can be carried out by an assistant or a colleague where time spent on various different activities are generally categorized under various heads. Such recording of activity logs can give a valuable insight into extra work time spent on unproductive activities and suitable corrective actions can be incorporated. Such time log or time motion research studies has been carried out previously in different hospital settings.(8–12)such as communication through a patient portal and administrative tasks, is increasing and contributing to burnout. The goal of this study was to assess time allocated by primary care physicians within the EHR as indicated by EHR user-event log data, both during clinic hours (defined as 8:00 am to 6:00 pm Monday through Friday

- **Planning every day in advance:** Begin each day with a 'to do' list. It is always good to have a master list, a monthly list, a weekly list and a daily list. Master list consists of a person's life-time goals, monthly list consists of the activities to be accomplished in the month, weekly list consists of the activities to be accomplished in the week and daily list consists of the activities to be accomplished in a particular day. It is always good to reassess the planning and see whether the daily, weekly and monthly lists are eventually taking a person closer to the final goal i.e the master list.

- **ABCDE technique:** This is about knowing and prioritizing what is important. This technique is all about rating the activities in order of priority, and doing the most important task first. Tasks can be grouped in five categories from A to E as follows:

  - A -very important work with huge consequences
  - B -important work with moderate consequences
  - C -good to do work but with no consequences
  - D -work that can be delegated to others
  - E -work that can be eliminated with no effect

- **Working out your individual/organizational goals:** Knowing the individual/organizational long-term goals will help a health manager plan better and focus on the activities that will help in achieving those goals. Knowing the final goal can be a determinant of how a health manger/professional spends his/her time efficiently towards the growth of himself/organization. Short term and medium-term goals can be incorporated to take the individual/organization closer towards the final goal.

- **Work Smarter, not Harder:** Proper time management does not require working harder for the results, it calls for smarter ways to pull off the required results. Health managers/professionals usually crib about being too busy nowadays and having limited time. Whereas they should concentrate on the results and work smartly towards their goals. It is not the quantity of work put in towards a particular goal, rather the quality that matters.

- **Delegate Responsibilities:** No matter how efficient a health manager is, he/she cannot perform all tasks on their own. It is important to find competent and reliable person and share the responsibilities. Rewards can be given on completion of delegated work in time. This will help in improving efficiency and productivity. In a retrospective cohort study carried out among primary care physicians in Wisconsin to assess workload using time- motion observations it was observed that the physicians spent nearly 6 hours on Electronic health records (EHR) in a day. Thus it was suggested that delegating such HER related work to other staff would reduce the burnout among the physicians.(8)such as communication through a patient portal and administrative tasks, is increasing and contributing to burnout. The goal of this study was to assess time allocated by primary care physicians within the EHR as indicated by EHR user-event log data, both during clinic hours (defined as 8:00 am to 6:00 pm Monday through Friday

- **Know Your Peak Times:** It is important for health managers/professionals to know what time of the day they feel the most energetic. As it is during this time that they are able to focus and concentrate better and hence must complete important projects at this time for better productivity.
- **Divide and Conquer:** Many a times health professionals/managers may get bogged down by bigger tasks/ projects. Such large projects can be easily dealt with by dividing such large projects into smaller tasks and completing one task at a time.

Management of Intrusions

Managing intrusions can go a long way in effective time management. Unnecessary or unproductive meetings can be avoided by healthcare professionals in managerial positions. Senior officials should allot specific time for meeting with outside visitors. Visitors must take prior appointment before the meeting. Senior officials can delegate certain meetings or tasks to juniors where their own presence is not necessary. Unnecessary paper work wherever possible can be kept to minimum. Keeping professional and social activities separate will keep more time for productive work.

Conclusion

Knowing how to manage time is essential for every health care professional. Without effective time management skills people tend to waste their valuable time on unimportant things and hence they do not achieve desirable results. Understanding the importance of time management skills and practicing the strategies in day-to-day life requires a great deal of determination from the individual to accomplish desirable results. Focusing on quality of work rather than quantity and completing one task at a time are important steps towards the larger goal.

Stress Management

Stress is the manner in which human beings react to various changes and situations in their lives. Stress cannot be avoided as it results from intricate interactions between an individual and his or her environment. (13) Though Stress is largely unavoidable, one can learn to manage Stress in order to lead a healthy life.

Stress is an inevitable part of one's life. While few stresses can be avoided and few have to be dealt with, overall balance of stress in one's life augurs well for the overall development of an individual. Different people experience stress in various different ways. The reaction is generally based on one's perception of any given situation. Stress is generally of two types; distress and eustress. A "negative" outlook towards any situation or event brings about the more common form of stress known as distress. On the other hand having a "positive" view of any situation results into eustress also known as the good stress. (14)

Due to the prolonged working hours, dealing with patients's life and death and the constant juggle between personal and professional lives; health care professionals are under constant stress. Right from the very beginning of the medical career where the curriculum is highly demanding, followed by the gruelling post graduate entrance examinations and then eventually searching for job or settling down; all these circumstances take a heavy toll on health care professionals.(15) It has been observed that stress among medical professionals at an early stage of their career such as during medical schools to a large extent determines the stress associated later with their profession and job satisfaction.(16,17) Hence stress management in the naïve years of medical college becomes of extreme importance.

Types of Stressors (18)

Any event or situation that induces stress is referred to as a "stressor". However, what one person finds stressful may not be the same for another. Being invited to attend a social event, for example, can cause discomfort for someone who believes they lack the requisite social skills to fit in, while another person who is at ease in social settings may not feel the same.

Stressors could be of varied forms and can come from different domains such as: (13,19)

1. Academic stressors which are the most commonly observed stressor amongst medical students. (20–23) there is a growing concern about stress during undergraduate medical training. The objectives of our study were to assess perceived stress among undergraduate medical students and to find out academic factors as determinants. A cross-sectional, questionnaire-based survey was carried out among undergraduate medical students of R. G. Kar Medical College, India, during July 2011-June 2012. Perceived stress was assessed using the Perceived Stress Scale-14. A 10-item questionnaire was used to assess academic sources of stress and their severity. The overall mean perceived stress score was 29.58 (standard deviation [SD] = 6.60 Few of the examples of academic stressors include vastness of curriculum, fear of failure in examination, competition with peers etc.

2. Social stressors could arise in the form of financial problems, job issues, expectations, family problems, social events, loneliness, job interviews, relationship issues etc.

3. Environmental stressors could vary from overcrowding, poverty, long queues in hospitals and other public places, traffic, noise, pollution, natural disasters etc.

4. Physiological stressors are in form of disease, injuries, pain, exposure to extremely hot or cold temperature, hormonal fluctuations etc.

5. Cognitive Stressors arise from the way one perceives a situation or what one expects out of the situation. Anxious thoughts, fearful anticipation and thinking negatively about a particular situation leads to increased stress.

Types of Stress

Acute stress

Acute stress is the most common form of stress. It is the human body's response to an upcoming challenge or an unexpected event. Normally, these occurrences of acute stress do not cause an individual any harm. They could even be beneficial to an individual's health. Such stressful situations make the human body and brain prepared to react in the most effective way to future stressful situations.

Generally, most people are aware of symptoms of acute stress. Examples of acute stress situations can be an important exam, a deadline, an upcoming performance etc. Acute stress lasts for a brief period, can crop up in anyone's life, and it is highly manageable.

Episodic acute stress

When an individual has repeated episodes of acute stress, this is known as episodic acute stress. This may occur if one is often nervous and concerned about events that one believes may occur. One may feel as though their life is in disarray and that they are going from one crisis to the next.

Persons experiencing episodic acute stress may feel like they are always under pressure and they would always be filled with negative energy. These people are constantly worried about negative things that could happen, and they are often rushed and impatient with so many demands on their time, all of which may lead to episodic acute stress. People who are experiencing such stress reactions are often over aroused, irritable, nervous, and tense.

Chronic stress

Chronic stress is a form of stress that develops over time as a result of prolonged emotional pressure. A demanding work, an unstable family situation, or financial difficulties are few of the precursors leading to chronic stress. It is the stress of never-ending demands and pressures which keep coming back like a vicious cycle.

Even if people become used to chronic stress and believe they no longer perceive it, it has a negative impact on their relationships and wellbeing. If a person is experiencing high levels of stress for an extended period of time, professional support is must. A mental health professional, such as a psychologist or counsellor, can assist in identifying such behaviours and situations that contribute to high stress and assist in making improvements to the situations that are within control.

Effects of Stress (18)

During stress, the human body reacts in a particular way. The Stress response could be in form of emotional, psychological, behavioral or physical manifestations.

Emotional response – This can manifest in form of anger, fear, impatience, worry, frustration, crying, guilt, unhappiness etc.

Psychological response – This can manifest in form of loss of wit, lack of focus, low self-esteem, forgetfulness, repetitive thoughts, lack of motivation etc.

Behavioral response – This can be observed in form of nervous tendencies, frequent mood swings, change in appetite, abuse others or abuse self, overtly aggressive or subdued behaviour, loss of libido, increase in alcohol consumption, increase in smoking etc.

Physical manifestations- This can be observed in form of bodyache, easy fatiguability, sweating, stuttering, palpitation, trembling, indigestion, insomnia, hypertension etc.

Stress Management Strategies

Stress management strategies are intended to keep stress levels in a healthy range. Good lifestyle choices will help to relieve stress and increase the chances of living a healthy life for prolonged period of time. Following are some evidence-based stress management techniques:

Progressive Muscle Relaxation (Pmr)

American physician Edmund Jacobson in the early 1920s developed a technique for reducing stress and anxiety known as Progressive muscle relaxation (PMR). This is a technique designed to relax one's body and mind by progressively tensing and relaxing of the muscle groups throughout the entire body. According to Jacobson, as stress and anxiety leads to tightening up of muscles, anxiety and stress can be reduced by learning how to relax the muscular tension.

This procedure is easy to understand and perform, also there are trained professionals who teach this procedure to individuals. This procedure can be performed over 2-3 sessions daily with each session spanning for 15-20 minutes.

Method: An individual can comfortably sit/lie down in a quiet place with eyes closed. Procedure begins by taking a few deep breaths. Then there is progressive tensing and relaxing of the various muscle groups over the legs, abdomen, chest, arms and face. The individual places a pressure in a given muscle group deliberately for about 10 seconds and then releases it for 20 seconds prior to proceeding with any successive muscle group. An individual is expected to focus and differentiate the different feeling at the time of tension and relaxation of muscle groups.

PMR has been used successfully to reduce Stress and fatigue and improving coping strategies among Intensive care unit nurses.(24) In a study done among medical students in Germany, it was observed that on offering an elective course in PMR, there was significant reduction in stress and burnout associated anxiety among the participating medical students.(25)

Biofeedback

Biofeedback is a feedback process that guides individuals to adjust their physiological behaviour in order to improve their health and performance. Brainwaves, heart function, breathing, muscle movement, and skin temperature are monitored using various instruments. These instruments record these physiological activities and send feedback to the user.

Method: This technique requires training in presence of a trained biofeedback therapist. The therapists work with their patients to discuss how to use different biofeedback devices to read and react to physiological details about their bodies. Generally, sessions are planned over a period of 3-6 months. After continuous practice, patients are able to take control of heart rate, blood pressure and other physiological functions.

In previous research conducted amongst healthcare providers, biofeedback tool was associated with a significant decline in stress. (26,27) In various studies conducted amongst nurses it was observed that biofeedback assisted mediation programs were associated with a decline in stress amongst the nurses. (28,29)

Diaphragmatic Breathing

Diaphragmatic breathing also known as deep breathing or abdominal breathing or belly breathing is a natural act of breathing which has been used as a means of relaxation instinctively. It is an act of breathing which involves extension of the abdomen rather than the chest. This technique has been an integral part of yoga and is currently incorporated in numerous relaxation programs.

During anxiety and stress, our breathing becomes shallower. Diaphragmatic breathing is a manipulation of breath movement which has been devised as an apt answer to this physiological change. This procedure is easy to understand and perform, also there are trained professionals who teach this procedure to individuals either manually or by means of audio or video.

Method - An individual can comfortably sit/lie down in a quiet place. Then take deep and relaxing breaths in and out to achieve a slow and steady breath. Then keeping one arm over chest and another over abdomen, perform slow deep breaths with expansion of the abdomen. This technique can be practiced for several sessions in a day with each session spanning over a few minutes.

In a quasi-experimental study conducted amongst nurses in Wuhan during the COVID-19 outbreak it was observed that Diaphragmatic breathing is very effective for improving the sleep quality and reducing anxiety. (30)

In various studies conducted amongst medical students, the students have reported decreased anxiety, nervousness, concentration loss and improved positive well-being using the deep breathing technique. (31,32)

Cognitive Behavioral Therapy (Cbt)

Cognitive Behaviour Therapy is a technique which looks at the link between thoughts, feelings and behaviour and assists individuals to find new ways to behave by changing their thought patterns. CBT is based on the idea that how we think about and view life events has an impact on how we act and, eventually, how we feel. CBT is a problem-specific, goal-oriented strategy that requires the individual's active participation to be effective.

Method: CBT is a clinical strategy that includes evaluation methods, cognitive and behavioural treatment approaches, and coordination between the clinician and the patient. Replacing irrational, counter-factual assumptions of the patient with more accurate and beneficial ones by the clinician is known as cognitive restructuring. This is accomplished by assisting the patient in becoming conscious of negative thought patterns, learning to challenge them, and replacing them with life-enhancing positive thought process and beliefs.

In various studies conducted amongst medical students, CBT came across as an efficient treatment for anxiety, hardiness, self-efficacy, and maladaptive perfectionism. (33–36)hardiness, and self-efficacy in female students of Birjand University of Medical Sciences.\n\nMATERIALS AND METHODS:\nThis was an interventional study. A sample of 30 participants were selected through the available sampling method and randomly assigned into experimental (CBT

Previous research have suggested that CBT can be very effective in reducing the burnout amongst the nurses, improving their mental health status, promoting healthy lifestyle beliefs and job satisfaction. (37–40)

Guided Imagery (Gi)

This is a technique which utilizes the power of mind, memory or imagination to create a sense of relaxation.

Method: This technique requires training by a trained professional by an audio, video or written script. Find a comfortable place and close your eyes. Think of a peaceful place where you would feel relaxed such as beach, hill station, nature, home etc. Take a moment to bring this place to your mind. Notice in that place whether you are alone or others are also present. Notice what dress you are wearing, different colours, objects, any pleasant smell. Desribe your skin coming in contact with any substance, any taste and how do you feel etc. The aim of the GI facilitator is to help the subject interact with his or her own imagination, which are a reflection of his or her particular health or life problems, in order to create health-promoting behaviour changes, or direct physiologic changes. The eventual aim to make the subject feel physically and emotionally relaxed.

Various studies conducted among health care professionals suggest that Guided imagery can be used as an important tool in reducing stress and anxiety, and increasing empathy and self-efficacy. (41,42)

Conclusion

There are many advantages from managing stress, such as an increase in focus, a decrease in anxiety, better health etc. Most significantly, stress management programmes empower an individual with a sense of control, which leads to increased self-esteem, reduced depression risk, and a better quality of life.

The aim of stress management programmes is to help health care professionals and medical students improve the ability to react to stressful incidents in a meaningful and productive manner. Stress-management interventions need to become more systematic and attend to the prevalent stressors in the work atmosphere to achieve a positive outcome. Individuals would be more adept at managing and handling challenging stressful life experiences if a robust stress management programme is implemented in the formative parts of their career. Rather than avoiding stressful circumstances, confronting them should be encouraged in the early part of their career.

Although teaching the medical students, staff and healthcare professionals stress-management skills is important and beneficial, it only addresses part of the issue. Both individual and organization-level factors should be given due importance. Many factors contribute to stress and time management issues, and resolving them normally necessitates the use of more than one strategy. One of the most significant advantages of time management and stress management is the eventual sense of control it provides to an individual.

References

1. Khatib ASA. Time Management and Its Relation To Students' Stress, Gender and Academic Achievement Among Sample of Students at Al Ain University of Science and Technology, UAE. Int J Bus Soc Res. 2014 May 20;4(5):47–58.

2. Macan TH, Shahani C, Dipboye RL, Phillips AP. College students' time management: Correlations with academic performance and stress. J Educ Psychol. 1990;82(4):760–8.

3. Brunicardi FC, Hobson FL. Time management: a review for physicians. J Natl Med Assoc. 1996 Sep;88(9):581–7.

4. Tracy B. Time management. New York: American Management Association; 2014. 104 p. (The Brian Tracy success library).

5. Harvey HB, Sotardi ST. The Pareto Principle. J Am Coll Radiol. 2018 Jun 1;15(6):931.

6. Tracy B. Eat that frog. 3rd ed. Berrett-Koehler; 2017.

7. Brannon LA, Hershberger PJ, Brock TC. Timeless demonstrations of Parkinson's first law. Psychon Bull Rev. 1999 Mar 1;6(1):148–56.

8. Arndt BG, Beasley JW, Watkinson MD, Temte JL, Tuan W-J, Sinsky CA, et al. Tethered to the EHR: Primary Care Physician Workload Assessment Using EHR Event Log Data and Time-Motion Observations. Ann Fam Med. 2017 Sep;15(5):419–26.

9. Despins LA, Kim JH, Deroche C, Song X. Factors Influencing How Intensive Care Unit Nurses Allocate Their Time. West J Nurs Res. 2019 Nov 1;41(11):1551–75.

10. Hripcsak G, Vawdrey DK, Fred MR, Bostwick SB. Use of electronic clinical documentation: time spent and team interactions. J Am Med Inform Assoc JAMIA. 2011;18(2):112–7.

11. Tai-Seale M, Olson CW, Li J, Chan AS, Morikawa C, Durbin M, et al. THE PRACTICE OF MEDICINE. Health Aff Proj Hope. 2017 Apr 1;36(4):655–62.

12. Marc Overhage J, McCallie Jr D. Physician Time Spent Using the Electronic Health Record During Outpatient Encounters. Ann Intern Med [Internet]. 2020 Jan 14 [cited 2021 Apr 22]; Available from: https://www.acpjournals.org/doi/abs/10.7326/M18-3684

13. Lin N, Ensel WM. Life Stress and Health: Stressors and Resources. Am Sociol Rev. 1989;54(3):382–99.

14. Parker KN, Ragsdale JM. Effects of Distress and Eustress on Changes in Fatigue from Waking to Working. Appl Psychol Health Well-Being. 2015;7(3):293–315.

15. Amr M, El Gilany AH, El-Hawary A. Does Gender Predict Medical Students' Stress in Mansoura, Egypt? Med Educ Online. 2008 Dec;13(1):4481.

16. Shaikh BT, Kahloon A, Kazmi M, Khalid H, Nawaz K, Khan N, et al. Students, stress and coping strategies: a case of Pakistani medical school. Educ Health Abingdon Engl. 2004 Nov;17(3):346–53.

17. Rani DRE, Ebenezer DrBSI, Gunturu3 DrVV. A Study on Stress Levels among First Year Medical Students: A Cross Sectional Study. IOSR-JDMS. 15(5):35–9.

18. Kumar A, Rinwa P, Kaur G, Machawal L. Stress: Neurobiology, consequences and management. J Pharm Bioallied Sci. 2013;5(2):91–7.

19. Raitano RE, Kleiner BH. Stress management: stressors, diagnosis, and preventative measures. Manag Res News. 2004 Jan 1;27(4/5):32–8.

20. Chowdhury R, Mukherjee A, Mitra K, Naskar S, Karmakar PR, Lahiri SK. Perceived psychological stress among undergraduate medical students: Role of academic factors. Indian J Public Health. 2017 Mar;61(1):55–7.

21. Brahmbhatt KR, P NV, S PK, S J. Perceived stress and sources of stress among medical undergraduates in a private medical college in Mangalore, India. Int J Biomed Adv Res. 2013 Mar 1;4(2):128–36.

22. Shah M, Hasan S, Malik S, Sreeramareddy CT. Perceived Stress, Sources and Severity of Stress among medical undergraduates in a Pakistani Medical School. BMC Med Educ. 2010 Dec;10(1):2.

23. Shankar PR, Balasubramanium R, Ramireddy R, Diamante P, Barton B, Dwivedi NR. Stress and Coping Strategies among Premedical and Undergraduate Basic Science Medical Students in a Caribbean Medical School. Educ Med J [Internet]. 2014 Dec 1 [cited 2020 Aug 9];6(4). Available from: http://eduimed.usm.my/EIMJ20140604/EIMJ20140604_05.pdf

24. Ozgundondu B, Gok Metin Z. Effects of progressive muscle relaxation combined with music on stress, fatigue, and coping styles among intensive care nurses. Intensive Crit Care Nurs. 2019 Oct 1;54:54–63.

25. Wild K, Scholz M, Ropohl A, Bräuer L, Paulsen F, Burger PHM. Strategies against Burnout and Anxiety in Medical Education – Implementation and Evaluation of a New Course on Relaxation Techniques (Relacs) for Medical Students. PLoS ONE [Internet]. 2014 Dec 17 [cited 2021 Feb 21];9(12). Available from: https://www.ncbi.nlm.nih.gov/pmc/articles/PMC4269409/

26. Lemaire JB, Wallace JE, Lewin AM, de Grood J, Schaefer JP. The effect of a biofeedback-based stress management tool on physician stress: a randomized controlled clinical trial. Open Med. 2011 Oct 4;5(4):e154–65.

27. Dunham CM, Burger AL, Hileman BM, Chance EA. Learning receptive awareness via neurofeedback in stressed healthcare providers: a prospective pilot investigation. BMC Res Notes [Internet]. 2018 Sep 4 [cited 2021 Feb 21];11. Available from: https://www.ncbi.nlm.nih.gov/pmc/articles/PMC6123908/

28. Cutshall SM, Wentworth LJ, Wahner-Roedler DL, Vincent A, Schmidt JE, Loehrer LL, et al. Evaluation of a biofeedback-assisted meditation program as a stress management tool for hospital nurses: a pilot study. Explore N Y N. 2011 Apr;7(2):110–2.

29. Hsieh H-F, Huang I-C, Liu Y, Chen W-L, Lee Y-W, Hsu H-T. The Effects of Biofeedback Training and Smartphone-Delivered Biofeedback Training on Resilience, Occupational Stress, and Depressive Symptoms among Abused Psychiatric Nurses. Int J Environ Res Public Health. 2020 Apr 22;17(8).

30. Liu Y, Jiang T, Shi T, Liu Y, Liu X, Xu G, et al. The effectiveness of diaphragmatic breathing relaxation training for improving sleep quality among nursing staff during the COVID-19 outbreak: a before and after study. Sleep Med. 2021 Feb;78:8–14.

31. Paul G, Elam B, Verhulst SJ. A Longitudinal Study of Students' Perceptions of Using Deep Breathing Meditation to Reduce Testing Stresses. Teach Learn Med. 2007 Jun 19;19(3):287–92.

32. Bughi SA, Sumcad J, Bughi S. Effect of Brief Behavioral Intervention Program in Managing Stress in Medical Students from Two Southern California Universities. Med Educ Online. 2006 Dec;11(1):4593.

33. Sahranavard S, Esmaeili A, Salehiniya H, Behdani S. The effectiveness of group training of cognitive behavioral therapy-based stress management on anxiety, hardiness and self-efficacy in female medical students. J Educ Health Promot [Internet]. 2019 Feb 15 [cited 2021 Feb 21];8. Available from: https://www.ncbi.nlm.nih.gov/pmc/articles/PMC6432834/

34. Chand SP, Chibnall JT, Slavin SJ. Cognitive Behavioral Therapy for Maladaptive Perfectionism in Medical Students: A Preliminary Investigation. Acad Psychiatry. 2018 Feb 1;42(1):58–61.

35. Lattie EG, Kashima K, Duffecy JL. An open trial of internet-based cognitive behavioral therapy for first year medical students. Internet Interv [Internet]. 2019 Sep 4 [cited 2021 Feb 21];18. Available from: https://www.ncbi.nlm.nih.gov/pmc/articles/PMC6743024/

36. Lattie EG, Duffecy JL, Mohr DC, Kashima K. Development and Evaluation of an Online Mental Health Program for Medical Students. Acad Psychiatry J Am Assoc Dir Psychiatr Resid Train Assoc Acad Psychiatry. 2017 Oct;41(5):642–5.

37. Bagheri T, Fatemi MJ, Payandan H, Skandari A, Momeni M. The effects of stress-coping strategies and group cognitive-behavioral therapy on nurse burnout. Ann Burns Fire Disasters. 2019 Sep 30;32(3):184–9.

38. Sampson M, Melnyk BM, Hoying J. Intervention Effects of the MINDBODYSTRONG Cognitive Behavioral Skills Building Program on Newly Licensed Registered Nurses' Mental Health, Healthy Lifestyle Behaviors, and Job Satisfaction. JONA J Nurs Adm. 2019 Oct;49(10):487–95.

39. Shariatkhah J, Farajzadeh Z, Khazaee K. The Effects of Cognitive-Behavioral Stress Management on Nurses' Job Stress. Iran J Nurs Midwifery Res. 2017;22(5):398–402.

40. Fadaei MH, Torkaman M, Heydari N, Kamali M, Ghodsbin F. Cognitive Behavioral Therapy for Occupational Stress among the Intensive Care Unit Nurses. Indian J Occup Environ Med. 2020;24(3):178–82.

41. Rao N, Kemper KJ. The Feasibility and Effectiveness of Online Guided Imagery Training for Health Professionals. J Evid-Based Complement Altern Med. 2017 Jan;22(1):54–8.

42. Boehm LB, Tse AM. Application of Guided Imagery to Facilitate the Transition of New Graduate Registered Nurses. J Contin Educ Nurs. 2013 Mar;44(3):113–9.

CHAPTER 7

Quantitative and Qualitative Estimations of Healthcare Management

Dr Jarina Begum

Professor, Dept of Community Medicine

Great Eastern Medical School and Hospital, Srikakulam, AP.

INTRODUCTION

In today's world, the healthcare system is evolving, technology is advancing, and healthcare delivery is progressing as per the increasing demand to provide quality health care, which could be made available at affordable prices, accessible through all windows and acceptable by all. However, the health administers, policy makers and health professionals are struggling with limited resources, competitive health management system and progressive demand for positive health. Healthcare managers must, therefore, find ways to get excellent results from more limited resources.[1]

Healthcare management is exactly what the name implies. It's the overall management of a healthcare facility, such as a clinic or hospital. A healthcare manager is in charge of ensuring a healthcare facility is running as it should in terms of budget, the goals of the facility's practitioners and the needs of the community. The terms 'healthcare management' and 'healthcare administration' are often mistakenly used interchangeably, and many people believe they are the same thing. They are two different things. Healthcare management is in charge of the entire healthcare organisation while healthcare administration takes care of the staff and employees.[2]

In today's complex, shifting healthcare landscape, much more is required to truly manage population health in fulfillment of the triple aim — improving patient health, improving patient experience and reducing healthcare costs. The next evolution of population health management, referred as Population Health 2.0, will demand a greater focus on these three key truths:

- Data is the new currency
- Data enables smarter decisions in real time
- Data makes a care team more efficient[3]

Management Process

1. Scanning the object being managed, the influences that surround it and diagnosing present and future problems
2. Formulating those problems so as to assess their significance, and to define aim and objectives
3. Generating alternate means of meeting objectives, examining them and choosing between them
4. Obtaining resources necessary to implement the chosen means
5. Defining tasks in such a way as to make effective use of available skills
6. Developing and enlarging skills and capabilities
7. Motivating people to accept the objectives and to work towards them
8. Monitoring, control and evaluation so as to adapt the chosen means in accordance with experience[4]

Management Methods and Techniques

Methods Based on Behavioural Sciences[5]:

Organisational Design: It is a systematic process for establishing the principles and structures that guide a business or organisation toward achieving its goals. This work culture has four components leadership, decision making, people and system.[6] A poor organisational design leads to wastage of resources. The organisation should be set up in such a way that is appropriate to the goals to be achieved. For example, a health system should be able to service the health needs of the population and the technology used should be kept up to date by regular upgrades

Personnel Management

Personnel management is defined as an administrative specialisation that focuses on hiring and developing employees to become more valuable to the company. It is sometimes considered to be a sub-category of human resources that only focuses on administration.

The Process of Personnel Management

The following are the steps involved in the process of personnel management:

(a) Human resource planning and forecasting
(b) Recruitment
(c) Selection,
(d) Training and development
(e) Performance appraisal
(f) Promotion and demotion[7]

Human resource is the most important part of an organisation. Proper methods of selection, training, motivation, allotment of roles, incentives and avenues for professional advancement should be ensured.

Communication: Communication is the exchange of meanings between individuals through a common system of symbols.[8] Communication between various levels is essential functioning of the system. Doctor-patient, doctor-nurse, health ministry-doctors — measures should be taken to ensure that there is free communication at these levels.

Lacunae in the communication system results in

- Delayed reporting of events
- Delayed supply of drugs and other resources
- Decreased efficiency of organisational function

Information System

The five main components that must come together in order to produce an Information System are hardware, software, data, network, people and highlights the relationships among the components and activities of information systems. An efficient information system should be in place to manage all the data. There should be a system for effective collection, classification, storage, retrieval, transformation and display of data. The information system plays an important part in monitoring and evaluation of the health system.

Management by Objectives (MBO)

The term Management by Objectives was coined by Peter Drucker in 1954.

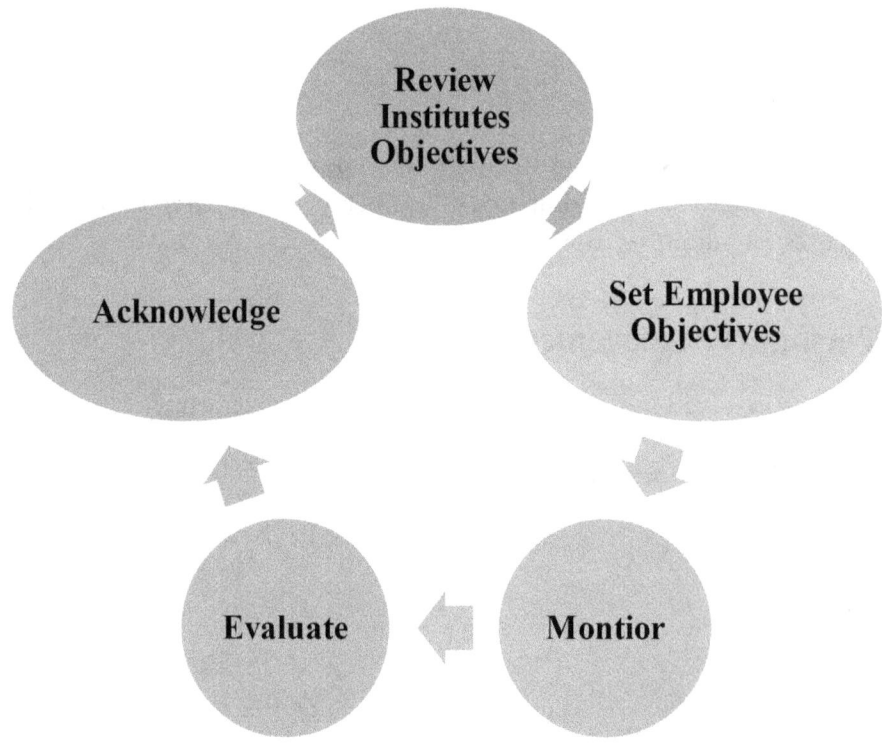

The process of setting up objectives in the organisation to give a sense of direction to the employees is known as Management by Objectives. It refers to the process of setting goals for the employees so that they know what they are supposed to do at the workplace. Management by Objectives defines roles and responsibilities for the employees and help them chalk out their future course of action in the organisation[9] In this, objectives are set for each unit and subunit of the system, and plans to attain these objectives are put forth and executed.

Quantitative Methods[10]

Quantitative methods are derived from the field of economics, operation research and budgeting. Some of these techniques have a great role in the management of health services:

Cost-Benefit Analysis

Cost benefit analysis (also known as a benefit cost analysis) is a process by which organisations can analyse decisions, systems or projects, or determine a value for intangibles. The model is built by identifying the benefits of an action as well as the associated costs, and subtracting the costs from benefits. When completed, a cost benefit analysis will yield concrete results that can be used to develop reasonable conclusions around the feasibility and/or advisability of a decision or situation. Cost-benefit analysis is a way to compare the costs and benefits of an intervention, where both are expressed in monetary units. The main drawback with this technique in health system is that the benefits in the health field, as a result of a particular programme, cannot always be expressed in monetary terms. We generally express the benefit in terms of births or deaths prevented, or illness avoided or overcome. Hence, the scope is limited.

Cost-effective Analysis

Cost-effectiveness analysis is a way to examine both the costs and health outcomes of one or more interventions. It compares an intervention to another intervention (or the status quo) by estimating how much it costs to gain a unit of a health outcome, like a life year gained or a death prevented.

Cost Accounting

Cost accounting is a method of accounting wherein all the costs involved in performing any process, project or product are noted and analysed. Such analysis helps the management in taking strategic decisions.[11]

It provides basic data on cost structure of any programme. Financial records are kept in a manner permitting costs to be associated with the purpose for which they are incurred. Cost accounting has three important purposes in health services: (a) cost control; (b) planning and allocation of people and financial resources; and (c) pricing of cost reimbursement.

Input-Output Analysis

Input–output analysis, economic analysis developed by the 20th century Russian-born US economist Wassily W Leontief, in which the interdependence of an economy's various productive sectors is observed by viewing the product of each industry both as a commodity demanded for final consumption and as a factor in the production of itself and other goods.[12] Input-output analysis is an economic technique. In the health field, "input" refers to all health service activities which consume resources (manpower, money, materials and time); and "output" refers to such useful outcomes as cases treated, lives saved or inoculations performed. An input output table shows how much of each "input" is needed to produce a unit amount of each "output". It enables calculations to be made of the effects of changing the inputs.

Model

The model is a basic concept of management science. It is an aid to understand how the factors in a situation affect one another. It is an abstraction of the reality, not the reality itself. The decision process includes the use of a model. "A problem-solving process used by an interdisciplinary team to develop mathematical models that represent simple-to-complex functional relationships and provide management with a basis for decision-making and a means of uncovering new problems for quantitative analysis".[13]

Systems Analysis

The purpose of systems analysis is to help the decision maker to choose an appropriate course of action by investigating his problem, searching out objectives, finding out alternative solutions, evaluation of the alternatives in terms of cost-effectiveness, re-examination of the objectives if necessary and finding the most cost-effective alternative.

Systems analysis is essentially finding the cost-effectiveness of the available alternatives. The system can be a hospital supply system, an information system, a total community health service system, an outpatient clinic or any other system with problems of management. A system may be made of independent subsystems.

Network Analysis

A network is a graphic plan of all events and activities to be completed in order to reach an end objective. It brings greater discipline in planning. The two common types of network technique are (a) PERT and (b) CPM.

PERT (Programme Evaluation and Review Technique) is a management technique which makes possible more detailed planning and more comprehensive supervision.

PERT is an appropriate technique which is used for the projects where the time required or needed to complete different activities are not known. PERT is majorly applied for scheduling, organisation and integration of different tasks within a project. It provides the blueprint of project and is efficient technique for project evaluation. Every homemaker who plans a meal so that each part of the menu is completed at the same time is using the basic technique of PERT. The essence of PERT is to construct an arrow diagram. The diagram represents the logical sequence in which events must take place. It is possible with such a diagram to calculate the time by which each activity must be completed, and to identify those activities that are critical. This simple technique provides a basic discipline by which all concerned in a project can know what is expected of them and to minimise any delays or crises in the implementation of the plan.

PERT is a useful management technique which can be applied to a great variety of projects.

Critical Path Method (CPM): The longest path of the network is called "critical path". If any activity along the critical path is delayed, the entire project will be delayed. CPM is a technique which is used for the projects where the time needed for completion of project is already known. It is majorly used for determining the approximate time within which a project can be completed. Critical path is the largest path in project management which always provide the minimum time taken for completion of project.[14]

Planning-Programming-Budgeting System (PPBS)

(PPBS) is a technique for optimising allocation of funds in the budget through exercise of proper choice among programmes which compete for limited resources. It involves three steps:

Planning: Identification of goals and objectives
Programming: Prioritising the goals
Budgeting: Allocation of funds[15]

The Planning-Programming-Budgeting System (PPBS) is primarily a system to help decision makers to allocate resources so that the available resources of an organisation are used in the most effective way in achieving its objectives. The PPBS does not call for changes in the existing organisation. It calls for grouping of activities into programmes related to each objective. Another approach is known as the 'Zero Budget Approach", i.e., all budgets start at zero and no one gets any budget that he cannot specifically justify on a year-to-year basis. With zero-based budgeting, you need to justify every expense before adding it to the official budget. The goal of zero-based budgeting is to reduce spending by looking at where costs can be cut.

Work Sampling

It is systematic observation and recording of activities of one or more individuals, carried out at predetermined or random intervals. The major parameters that are analysed are the type of activities performed and the time needed to do specified jobs.

Decision Making

Decision making is just like the basic discipline of differential diagnosis in medical practice. It is an adage that decisions should be made at the level where the best decisions can be made; it does not follow that the best decision is always made at the top of an organisation.

References

1. https://dl.uswr.ac.ir/bitstream/Hannan/130435/1/Yasar_A._Ozcan_PhD_Quantitative_Methods_in_Health_Care_Management_Techniques_and_Applications__2009.pdf

2. https://www.healthcare-management-degree.net/faq/what-is-healthcare-management/

3. https://hitconsultant.net/2014/07/07/future-of-population-health-management/

4. WHO. *Modern Management Methods and the Organization of Health Services*. Public Health papers 55, 1974.

5. https://pgblazer.com/management-methods-based-on-behavioural-sciences/

6. https://pingboard.com/blog/organizational-design-101-what-to-know-before-attempting-your-own/

7. https://cio-wiki.org/wiki/Personnel_Management#:~:text=Personnel%20management%20is%20defined%20as,that%20only%20focuses%20on%20administration.

8. GN Gordon. 'Communication'. *Encyclopedia Britannica*. 16 December 2020. https://www.britannica.com/topic/communication

9. https://www.managementstudyguide.com/management-by-objectives.htm

10. *Park's Textbook of Preventive and Social Medicine*, 25th ed, pp 934-35.

11. https://cleartax.in/s/cost-accounting

12. T Editors of Encyclopaedia. *Britannica*. 13 February 2020. *Input–output analysis. Encyclopedia Britannica*. https://www.britannica.com/topic/input-output-analysis

13. https://www.businessmanagementideas.com/essays/management-science-definition-characteristics-and-tools/9080

14. https://www.geeksforgeeks.org/difference-between-pert-and-cpm/

15. https://blog.forumias.com/what-is-planning-programming-and-budgeting-system-ppbs/

Chapter 8

Time Motion in Health care Management

Dr Rashmi Agarwalla

Assistant Professor, Dept. of Community and Family Medicine

All India Institute of Medical Sciences Guwahati

INTRODUCTION

Frederick Taylor (1856–1915) concluded after his research on inefficiencies in industrial processes that one of the biggest loss in any kind of processes was due to wastage of human effort. He contributed to the emerging "scientific management" field with his Time Study method aiming at reducing processes' times.[1]

Initially time studies were conducted by observing the time consumed by workers to accomplish a task. Taylor's disciples Frank and Lilian Gilbreth, later on expanded the method and focused on motion.[2] Time study, which initially originated by Taylor was mainly used for time measurement; and motion study, which was developed by the Gilbreth's, was largely used for improving methods, while one group saw time measurement as a means of determining the tasks done in a day, another group looked into motion study for determining a good method of doing work.[3] These two techniques, the time studies and the motion studies, were later on integrated and thus became one of the accepted methods in scientific management which is now known as the Time Motion Studies (TMS).[2] TMS is a methodology which ensures recording of time duration of every activity to establish work flow and ensure efficiency and effectiveness through the elimination of waste and simplification of work.

Use of Time Motion Studies

In 1914, the motion study technique was used by Gilberth for the assessment of inefficiencies in the healthcare industry.[1] Slowly health care managers and researchers started using TMS for assessing costs and inefficiencies in delivery of health care. Now TMS is widely used to conduct studies to assess quality in health care management and thereby contribute towards efficient and quality patient care.

Time-motion study is mainly used for two purposes:[3]

1. To assist in finding the most efficient method of doing work; and
2. To assist in training individuals to understand the meaning of time-motion importance, and when the training is carried out with sufficient thoroughness, to enable them to become proficient in applying time motion principles.

Some essential components of successful TMS are well trained manpower, who are well practiced and are quick on their feet and at the same time are not compromising on quality.

The following additional design and process elements as mentioned could contribute to a successful Time and Motion study:[4]

1. **Strategic evidence matters:** Choosing an appropriate study and design are crucial for scientifically robust evidence.
2. **Less is more.** Important Study variables must be carefully chosen to ensure that only the variables of utmost importance are included.
3. **Keep it simple.** The Case report form used by the observer must be user-friendly. The formats should be designed with the predicted chronological order of healthcare events and resource utilization of interest in mind, along with the awareness that observers are likely juggling a writing instrument, a stop-watch, and a CRF.
4. **Find the common ground.** Each task should be described on the Case Report Form clearly and in accurate form so as to ensure uniformity and common understanding. Definitions should be uniform and generation of good quality data should be of paramount importance for efficient data analysis.
5. **Invest in local leadership.** Investment should be made in local leadership and participating study site should offer local staff who are engaged and committed to the day-to-day management of the study.
6. **Training and Retraining should be done:** Training of the observers should be standardized across all participating centers to cross check inter-observer variability in stopwatch measurement.
7. **Knowing the team and collaborators:** At the beginning of each observation day, if feasible, it is suggested that observers meet the healthcare staff that will be providing care to the study subjects that day. This provides an opportunity for observers to pre-identify the role each healthcare staff plays on the care team. This familiarization can contribute directly to the accuracy of timings that need to be recorded by the observers.
8. **Data should not get cold:** Data should be processed immediately and should be communicated back to the observer within a reasonable recall period.
9. **Choose the right data analytic technique.** Data should be analyzed using appropriate statistical test and technique. Appropriate techniques may be used for adjusting for relevant co-variates. Time motion studies plays an important role in health care management of countries like India where many programs are running and there is concern regarding performance and time management of grass root level and frontline health workers. Many studies have been done to assess time utilization and work flow of these workers in various set ups. The technique has been utilized to see working of community health workers, pharmacists, nurses, working in vaccination process etc.[5,6,7,8,9]

Challenges for Time Motion Studies

Although time motion studies have been helpful in many aspects, they have certain limitations:

Time motion study is found to be not suitable for non-repetitive jobs and also it is not found suitable for jobs which are not standardized or indirect labor jobs.

It is less suitable for jobs conducted by automatic machines than in the jobs which are operator controlled.

Hawthorne effect could act as a major limitation in Time and Motion studies as observers could interfere with care patterns by their presence. Moving through time and space, while juggling a stopwatch, pen, and CRF, is indeed a challenge for the observers charged with the mandate to produce complete and high quality data.

Conclusion

A time motion study should ideally be complemented by qualitative enquiry to spot opportunities so as to reach conclusions which will help in getting the work done more efficiently.

References

1. Marcelo Lopetegui, MD, Po-Yin Yen, RN, PhD, Albert Lai, PhD, Joseph Jeffries, Peter Embi, MD, MS, and Philip Payne, PhD. Time Motion Studies in Healthcare: What are we talking about?. J Biomed Inform. 2014; 0:292–299.doi:10.1016/j.jbi.2014.02.017.

2. Baumgart A, Neuhauser D. Frank and Lillian Gilbreth: scientific management in the operating room. Qual Saf Health Care 2009;18:413–415.

3. Bhargo L, Mishra A, Agarwal AK. Time-Motion Study to Know: Efficiency and Effectiveness of Clinical Care is Essential to Hospital Function? Indian Journal of Community Medicine 2014;39(40):254-55.

4. Time and Motion studies, opportunities and challenges. Pharaphorum bringing healthcare together.2014. Available[internet].https://pharmaphorum.com/views-and-analysis/time-and-motion-studies-opportunities-and challenges/.[last accessed on 2nd Feb 2021].

5. Chebolu-Subramanian, Sule N, Sharma R, and Mistry N. A time motion study of community mental health workers in rural India. BMC Health Services Research 2019;19:878.

6. Fisher AM, Ding MQ, Hochheiser H, Douglas GP. Measuring time utilization of pharmacists in the Birmingham free clinic dispensary. BMC Health Serv Res. 2016;16:529.

7. Mokiou S, De Cock E, Standaert B. Workflow mapping for Paediatric vaccination process in the United Kingdom: a precursor of a time and motion (T & M) study. Value Health. 2014;17(7):582.

8. Tipping MD, Forth VE, O'Leary KJ, Malkenson DM, Magill DB, Englert K, et al. Where did the day go – a time-motion study of hospitalists. J Hosp Med. 2010;5(6):328.

9. Zheng K, Guo MH, Hanauer DA. Using the time and motion method to study clinical work processes and workflow: methodological inconsistencies and a call for standardized research. J Am Med Inform Assoc. 2011;18(5): 701–10.

Chapter 9

Overview of Health Administration

At the village, block, district, state and centre level in India

Dr Sumit Aggarwal, Dr Sivaraman Balaji, Dr J Madhumathi

Scientist, Epidemiology and Communicable Diseases Division

Indian Council of Medical Research-Headquarters, Ansari Nagar, New Delhi

Dr Yogita Bavaskar

Associate Professor, Department of Community Medicine

Jalgano Medical College, Jalgano, Maharashtra

INTRODUCTION

Health is an essential criterion for day-to-day activities of human life. Countries around the globe are striving to advance and expand their health care delivery services on a priority basis over the others. Ultimately, state or province authority has a responsibility for the health of its people. Several factors including the social, economic, political and environmental, impact the health care delivery system of countries, which influence their growth and development (Peabody et al, 2006). A health system is also referred to as a health care system that comprises society, organisation and resources that provide health care services to the people of that country. Although healthcare is a government affair in India, certain NGOs have also taken considerable efforts. Thus, since independence, India has developed an extensive health infrastructure including both public and private sector (Bajpai, 2014; Chokshi et al, 2016).

Most individuals and societies assumed that good health or wellness is the absence of disease. In contrast, health is a highly desirable state for all human being and individual perception. Wellness is the state in which a person function at an optimal level. In both developed and developing countries, the current aim is to reach the population with adequate healthcare services and secure an acceptable level of health through primary healthcare facilities Farklılıklar, 2018; Boruchovitch and Mednick, 2002, CDC, 2018). It constitutes the management sector and involves organisational matters. It operates in the context of the socioeconomic and political framework of the country. In India, there are five significant segments and agencies independent of each other by the technology applied for health and by the source of funds for the operation (Bajpai, 2014).

1. Public health sector provides health care through hospitals and monitors the national health
2. Private sectors deliver health service through various hospitals
3. Indigenous system of medicine by the Ministry of AYUSH
4. Voluntary health agencies include NGOs
5. National health programmes monitored by the union health ministry

WHO has identified the inequalities in access to health care among the people, especially in developing and under developing countries. Necessary actions must be taken to improve in these aspects, especially to evade discrimination. The current challenge for most countries is to reach their people with adequate health care services and ensure their utilisation (Donnell, 2007).

Healthcare Delivery System in India

India contains 31 states and seven union territories, where states are mainly independent, relating to delivering health care to the public. Each state deserves its organisation structure of health care delivery which is autonomous and independent of the central government. Making new or updating policies, preparation, supervisory, supporting, assessing and coordinating is carried out by the central government. The overall health system in India has three main components:

1. Central
2. State, and
3. Local or peripheral

At the Central Level

Union Ministry of Health and Family Welfare

The funding source for running public agencies is tax money; thus, these are accountable to the common public. In general, the public sector comprises both official and charitable agencies organized at several levels. A cabinet minister heads the Union Ministry of Health and Family Welfare (MoHFW). Besides, there will be a minister of state, and occasionally a deputy health minister. Though these are political posts, they have a dual role in both political and administration. The ministry could undertake any public or private agencies/organization for several reasons. For instance, Department of AIDS Control has been merged with the Department of Health & Family Welfare in 2014 and now known as the National AIDS Control Organization (NACO). As per the amendment in the allocation of business rules by cabinet secretariat's notification department of AYUSH (which was part of MoHFW earlier) has been made Ministry of Ayurveda, Yoga and Naturopathy, Unani, Siddha and Homeopathy (AYUSH) with focused attention on the development of education and research in ayurveda, yoga and naturopathy, unani, siddha and homoeopathy systems (Shankar, 2017). Organisation structure for the Ministry of Health and Family Welfare at the institutional level is given in Figure 1. Presently, MoHFW comprise of two separate departments and headed by different secretaries to the Government of India:

1. Department of Health and Family Welfare
2. Department of Health Research

In addition to these departments, Directorate General of Health Services (DGHS) is an independent body coming under the Department of Health & Family Welfare. This has secondary offices that spread all over the country at each state. The central role of DGHS is to provide technical advice on all medical and public health stuff, which is highly important for the implementation of several Health Services initiated by MoHFW. In India, the constitutional provisions on the subject of the distribution of legislative powers between the central and the states are demarcated in several articles where Articles 245 and 246 are more critical incidentally being specific. The Seventh Schedule to the Constitution of India clearly shows and stipulates distribution of authorities and functions between the Centre and states which contains three lists; i.e. (1) Union List, (2) State List and (3) Concurrent List.

Union List

The union list contains the 100 numbered items listed in the Seventh Schedule to India's Constitution. The central government or Indian Parliament deserves exclusive power to legislate on matters relating to these items.

1. International health relations and administration of port quarantine.
2. Administration of central institutes such as All India Institute of Hygiene and Public Health, Kolkata.
3. Research promotion through various research centres.
4. Regulation and development of medical, pharmaceutical, dental and nursing professions.
5. Establishment and maintenance of drug standards.
6. Census and collection and publication of other statistical data.
7. Immigration and emigration.
8. Central government health schemes.
9. Regulation of labour in the working of mines and oil fields.
10. Organising states and other ministries for the promotion of health.
11. Development of teaching material regarding health for making health awareness through central health education bureau.
12. Collection, compilation, analysis, evaluation and dissemination of information through the Central Bureau of Health Intelligence.
13. Implementation, operation and evaluation of various national health programmes.
14. Consider and recommend broad outlines of policy concerning health issues like environment hygiene, nutrition, and health education.
15. To make proposals for legislation relating to medical and public health matters.
16. To make recommendations to the central government regarding the distribution of grants-in-aid.
17. To establish any organisation or organisations invested with appropriate functions for promoting and maintaining cooperation between the central and state health administration.

State List

The state list contains the list of 61 numbered items which is listed in the Schedule Seven to the Constitution of India. The state governments have exclusive authority to establish on matters relating to public health and sanitation, and hospitals and dispensaries.

Concurrent List

There are 52 items currently added to this concurrent list. Both the central and state government have the responsibility in performing the items listed in the concurrent list;

1. Prevention and extension of communicable diseases
2. Prevention of adulteration of food kinds of stuff
3. Control of drugs and poisons
4. Vital statistics
5. Labour welfare
6. Ports other than significant
7. Economic and social planning
8. Population control and family planning

At the State Level

State Health Administration

As per the Montague-Chelmsford reforms, all India states got autonomy from central government related to the public health in 1919. As a result, all states formed the basic system of public health organization in 1920-1921. Further, the Government of India Act, 1935 provided more independence to the states. As per this law, the state deserves the decisive authority for health services operating within its jurisdiction. In all the states, the management sector comprises the State Ministry of Health and a Directorate of Health, but few states have a single ministry for both sectors. The primary responsibility for providing health services to all people lies with the State Health Department, with local health organisations' assistance wherever they exist, e.g. corporations, municipalities, panchayati raj, ad-hoc statutory bodies the Mines Board of Health, employees, State Insurance Corporation and so on. At the state level, the administrative machinery of the government is headed by the governor. According to Article Number 163 of the Constitution, a council of ministers with the chief minister as its head to aid and advise the governor. The governor amongst the minister allocates the state's government (viz law and order administration, local government, public works, irrigation, health education, cooperation, etc) following the provisions contained is Article 166(3) of the Constitution. Administrative structure for the state ministry of health and medical education and research is provided in the Figure 2.

Organisation of the State Health Department

Political Head: State Department of Health and Family Welfare, headed by the State Minister of Health and Family Welfare. One has to bear responsibility for formulating policies and monitoring the implementation of these policies and programmes. The health minister has to perform both types of activities, viz., political and administrative (Figure 2).

Administration Head: In order to maintain the policies framed by the political heads and to supervise their implementation and executive, the state administration has an office, which is known as the state secretariat. The word 'secretariat' denotes the complex of departments which vary among each state. The health department's secretariat is a vital place of the State Ministry of Health which a secretary controls. Several additional secretaries, deputy secretaries, and a large administrative staff will assist the secretary. Although there are no strict rules, most states follow two broader divisions to the health.

1. **The Department of Public Health:** It consists of the directorate of medical and rural health services, Directorate of Public Health, Directorate of Health and Family Welfare, Directorate of Drugs Control, Directorate of Health Transport, State Health Mission and Preventive Medicine are the critical technical directorates to the state government on all matters related to public health.

2. **The Department of Medical Education and Research:** This other directorate namely Directorate of Medical Education and research, depends upon the state's decision. It controls medical and paramedical colleges and related things in that particular state. Rarely, some states may have a discrete ministry to administrate medical education and research.

Technical Head: Under the state secretariat, various administrative departments are working. These departments are mostly controlled by specialists with the supervision, coordination, and control of the state government's policy. The Director of Health Services is the principal technical consultant to the state government on all matters relating to medicine and public health. Additionally, the director is accountable for the organisation and direction of all health activities. He is assisted by deputies and assistants of various fields where they may be of two categories, either **regional or functional.** The *regional director* holds the authority to inspects all the divisions of public health that fall under their jurisdiction, regardless of their field. In contrast, the *functional directors* are generally specialists in a specific division of public health, namely mother and child health, family planning, nutrition, tuberculosis, leprosy, health education, etc.

At The District Level

India has a diverse healthcare organisation structure, inclusive of public and private healthcare service providers. Majority of the private health sectors are focused on the urban regions and delivering secondary and tertiary healthcare services. However, the public healthcare organisation in rural parts has been established as a three-tier system, mostly classified based on the population norms developed by the Shrivastav Committee's recommendations in 1975. Each of these three systems is monitored by a higher level to which the patient is referred. The perception of primary healthcare began in 1978, after an international conference heled in ALMA ATA, USSR. This approach is mainly founded on social equity principles, nationwide coverage, self-reliance, inter-sectoral coordination, and health programmes to pursue common health goals. This is also demarcated as "health by the people, and placing people's health in people's hand" it is defined in the following way: "Primary health care is essential health care made universally accessible to individuals and acceptable to them, through full participation and at a cost the community and country can afford" (Lahariya et al, 2020). Flow chart explain the detailed political and administrative structure of both general and health administration at district level is given as Figure 3.

Levels of Healthcare in India

Primary Healthcare

This is the primary level of interaction between the individual and the health system. Mostly, all of the health complaints and problems can be acceptably dealt at this level. Provided at the PHC, SC (sub centre).

Village Level

The below-mentioned schemes are functioning at the village level:

1. Village health guides scheme
2. Training of local dais (past procedure)
3. ICDS scheme

Sub-centre Level

This is the peripheral outpost of the existing health care delivery system in rural areas. They are operated differently based on the population of the region. For instance, there is a one sub-centre for every 5,000 populations in typical landscape whereas one for every 3000 populations in hilly tribal and backward areas (Bashar and Goel, 2017). This healthcare sector forms the primary connection point between the primary health-care system and the community. Each SC must be operated by as a minimum of one auxiliary nurse midwife (ANM)/female health worker and one male health worker. Additionally, as per the National Rural Health Mission (NRHM), the SC can recruit one more ANM on a contract basis. SCs are assigned tasks relating to interpersonal communication to bring about behavioural change and provide services concerning maternal and child health, family welfare, nutrition, immunization, diarrhoea control, and communicable diseases programs. The MoHFW provides complete central support to all the country's SCs since April 2002 in the form of financial support, rental and contingencies, and medications and equipment (Pyone et al, 2019).

Primary Health Centre (PHC)

PHC is a primary connection point between the village people and the medical officer. Similar to SC, PHCs are established in different regions based on population strength. These are operated in a natural area with 30,000 people and hilly/difficult to reach/tribal areas with 20,000. PHCs were envisioned to deliver combined curative and preventive health care to the rural population, emphasising the preventive and promotive aspects of health care (Lahariya, 2020; Sriram, 2018). PHCs are mostly formed and maintained by the state governments and comes under the Minimum Needs Program (MNP)/Basic Minimum Services (BMS) Program. PHC must be supervised by the medical officer who should be supported by a maximum of 14 paramedical and other staff. Additionally, as per NRHM, there is a provision for two more staff nurses at PHCs on a contract basis. In general, It serves as a recommendation unit for five-six SCs and has a minimum of four-six beds for inpatients. The activities of PHCs involve healthcare promotion and curative services.

Secondary Healthcare

These are the second tier of the healthcare system, where patients from PHCs are referred to specialists for higher treatment options. In India, the facility for secondary healthcare is provided in district hospitals and community health centre at the block level. This level attends more complex health-associated problems (Ramani and Sivakami, 2019).

Community Health Centers (CHCs)

CHCs are developed and sustained by the state government under the MNP/BMS programme. In general, CHCs are established for normal landscape area with a population of 1,20,000 people and in hilly/difficult to reach/tribal areas with a population of 80 000. CHCs have 30 beds for inpatients equipped with x-ray labour room, laboratory and operation theatre facility. CHCs must be staffed by four medical experts, such as the surgeon, physician, gynecologist/obstetrician and paediatrician. Besides, this should be supported by at least 21 paramedical and other staff. It serves as a referral centre for PHCs within the block and provides facilities for obstetric care and specialist consultations (Sodani and Sharma, 2011).

Any existing facility to be declared as a fully operational first referral unit (FRU) that must be prepared to deliver continuous services for emergency obstetric and newborn care, in addition to all emergencies. These are the three essential determinants for FRU: (1) emergency obstetric care including surgical interventions such as caesarean sections; (2) care for small and sick newborns; and (3) blood storage facility on a 24-hour basis (Raman et al, 2009).

Tertiary Health Care

This is the third level of India's health system, in which specialised consultative care is delivered at the super speciality and medical college hospitals based on the recommendation from primary and secondary medical care centres (Bajpai, 2014). Specialized Intensive Care Units, progressive diagnostic support services and dedicated medical personnel are critical features of tertiary health care. Tertiary care service is generally delivered by medical colleges and advanced medical research institutes. This level offers super speciality care provided by the regional and central level institution.

References

1. V Bajpai. 'The Challenges Confronting Public Hospitals in India, Their Origins, and Possible Solutions'. *Advances in Public Health*, 2014.

2. MA Bashar, & S Goel. 'Are Our Subcenters Equipped Enough to Provide Primary Health Care to the Community: A Study to Explore the Gaps in Workforce and Infrastructure in the Subcenters from North India'. *Journal of Family Medicine and Primary Care*, 6(2), p 208. 2017.

3. E Boruchovitch, and BR Mednick. 'The Meaning of Health and Illness: Some Considerations for Health Psychology'. *Psico-USF*, 7(2), pp 175-83. 2002.

4. CDC, 'Well Being Concept'. 2020. https://www.cdc.gov/hrqol/wellbeing.htm.

5. M Chokshi, B Patil, R Khanna, SB Neogi, J Sharma, VK Paul, and S Zodpey. 'Health Systems in India'. *Journal of Perinatology*, 36(3), pp. S9-S12. 2016.

6. A Farklılıklar. 'Differences in the Perception of Health among the Urban Poor Living in Two Squatter House Neighbourhoods in Ankara'. *Mediterranean Journal of Humanities*, pp 309-33. 2018.

7. C Lahariya. 'Health & Wellness Centers to Strengthen Primary Health Care in India: Concept, Progress and Ways Forward'. *The Indian Journal of Pediatrics*, pp 1-14. 2020.

8. JW Peabody, MM Taguiwalo, DA Robalino, and J Frenk. 'Improving the Quality of Care in Developing Countries'. 2006.

9. Thidar Pyone, Shilpa Karvande, Somasundari Gopalakrishnan, Vidula Purohit, Sarah Nelson, Subha Sri Balakrishnan, Nerges Mistry, and Matthews Mathai. 'Factors Governing the Performance of Auxiliary Nurse Midwives in India: A Study in Pune District.' *PloS one* 14, no 12: e0226831. 2019.

10. P Raman, B Sharma, D Mavalankar, and M Upadhyaya. 'Assessing the Regional and District Capacity for Operationalizing Emergency Obstetric Care Through First Referral Units in Gujarat'. 2009.

11. S Ramani, and M Sivakami. 'Community Perspectives on Primary Health Centers in Rural Maharashtra: What Can we Learn for Policy?' *Journal of Family Medicine and Primary Care*, 8(9), p 2837. 2019.

12. D Shankar, and B Patwardhan. 'AYUSH for New India: Vision and Strategy'. *Journal of Ayurveda and Integrative Medicine*, 8(3), p 137. 2017.

13. D Shankar, and B Patwardhan. 'AYUSH for New India: Vision and Strategy'. *Journal of Ayurveda and Integrative Medicine*, 8(3), p 137. 2017.

14. PR Sodani and K Sharma. 'Assessing Indian Public Health Standards for Community Health Centers: A Case Study with Special Reference to Essential Newborn Care Services'. *Indian Journal of Public Health*, 55(4), p 260. 2011.

15. S Sriram. 'Availability of Infrastructure and Manpower for Primary Health Centers in a District in Andhra Pradesh, India'. *Journal of Family Medicine and Primary Care*, 7(6), p 1256. 2018.

16. WHO. 'A Vision for Primary Health Care in the 21st Century'. *UNICEF*. 2018.

Chapter 10

Medical Audit

Dr Vidisha Vallabh

Assistant Professor, Department of Community Medicine

HIMS, SRH University, Dehradun, Uttarakhand

Dr Deep Shikha

Associate Professor, Department of Community Medicine

HIMS, SRH University, Dehradun, Uttarakhand

WHAT IS AUDIT?

The term audit (Latin: audire) which means to hear (an official account) in modern world refers to "to make an official examination of the accounts of a business and produce a report" and is not limited to the world of finance any more, involving the examination of records or financial accounts to check their accuracy (1,2). In the healthcare sector, medical auditing, is a relatively new field that examines and reviews medical records, to ensure that the healthcare providers and facilities are in compliance with the pre-set standards (3).

History of Medical Audit

Medical audit also known as clinical audit is a means to improve the quality of patient care. It was born out of the need to take care of people and tracing its origins is an arduous task. Nevertheless, the recorded mentions of audit have been found as early as 1750 BC. Another well-known incident is the auditing by Florence Nightingale during the Crimean War of 1835-55, which reduced the mortality among the soldiers by half (4,5). In modern medicine, medical audits were formally started in 1920s and by 1950s standardised formats were available. Ernest Codman, an orthopedic surgeon and Avedis Donabedian, who gave the oft quoted model for quality of care have been regarded as the fore-fathers of medical audit (6–8). A standardised clinical audit was introduced by National Health Services (UK) as a part of professional health care in 1993. This soon led to development and implementation of standards in health care worldwide (7).

Meaning of Medical Audit

"Clinical (or medical) audit is a quality improvement process that seeks to improve patient care and outcomes through systematic review of care against explicit criteria and the implementation of change. Aspects of the structure, process and outcomes of care are selected and systematically evaluated against explicit criteria.

Where indicated changes are implemented at an individual, team or service level and further monitoring is used to confirm improvement in healthcare delivery" (9–11).

Clinical audit is used routinely to assess quality of care in developed countries. Developing nations like India are still struggling to provide basic healthcare to its people, the dream of a nation-wide audit data system is a far-fetched dream (12). Though they look the same, medical audit is quite different from research and data collection. Research is systematic investigation that may involve experiments and usually results in unearthing new information about patient treatment. Audit, on the other hand, systematically reviews current practices in healthcare without any experiments to ascertain the best practices and standards in healthcare. It can act as a precursor for research by unearthing the deficient areas in patient care. Similarly, data collection is concerned with general data whereas audit focuses on a specific process or structure and suggests changes in them which are again reassessed after sometime (2, 7, 9, 13).

Medical audit, therefore, systematically analyses the current practices in medicine, including all aspects of patient care like diagnosis, treatment and resourcefulness and makes a quantifiable comparison against the pre-set standards in healthcare. The suggestions from this audit are used to improve the quality of patient care (11,14,15).

The terms medical and clinal audit will be used interchangeably in the chapter, although clinical audit has multiple components related to patients, education and training, health care delivery, resources for health, working relationships, and so on (16).

Why Do We Need Medical Audit?

Audit critically analyses the current practices in healthcare by the healthcare provider and shows them the gaps where improvement can be done. It is a planned programme which objectively monitors and evaluates the clinical performance of all practitioners, which identifies scopes for improvement, and provides mechanism through which action is taken to make and sustain those improvements (17).

The main motives of a healthcare establishment, behind a medical audit can be professional (to identify own deficiencies and correct them), social (safeguard patients from harmful practices) or pragmatic (provide best possible service to patients), financial (generate cost saving ideas) and educational. They can also gap the bridge of doctor-patient, doctor-nurse and nurse-patient communication and help in reducing wasteful activities (17–19).

Audit can help a healthcare provider ascertain:

1. Whether the quality of healthcare is meeting the desired standards
2. If the quality of health care has improved as compared to the previous audit
3. If there is a variation in quality of healthcare from national average
4. The degree of lacunae in their quality
5. The necessary suggestion to fill these lacunae
6. Protect against fraudulent claims and billing activity.
7. To stop the use of outdated or incorrect codes for procedures
8. To verify ICD-10-CM and electronic health record (EHR) meaningful use readiness

Hence, medical audit may be performed by the sole healthcare provider, by the team or institution that provides healthcare (internal audit), by external reviewers (external audit) (17, 20–22).

Methods of Audit

Information for audit can be collected from various sources (18, 23–28).

1. **Case Note Review:** Review of selected cases (eg. laparotomy, prescription writing, post-partum haemorrhage, cochlear implantation) have been known to reduce the complications in future cases. The aim is to establish facts and to look for adherence to policies and procedures or to discover deviations from it. This is the main method used in mortality and morbidity reviews.
2. **Semi-quantitative Studies:** If reviews are made on a considerable number of similar individual cases, (as described above), certain conclusions can be generalised based on the frequency of occurrences of certain events among the cases.
3. Analysis of routinely collected health service data
4. Population-based epidemiological studies/quantitative studies
5. Analysis of the appropriate use of investigations and therapies

The Audit Cycle

Steps of an auditing cycle are as follows:

Stage 1: **Planning for Audit:** Decide the topic, plan and train the team.

Stage 2: **Standard/Criteria Selection:** Determine the criteria for the current best practice.

Stage 3: **Data Collection and Measuring Performance:** Identify what data needs to be collected, how, and who is going to collect it. Decide whether the data will be collected prospectively or retrospectively and what sample size is needed. Analyse the data collected (actual performance within the department) with the set standard. Evaluate how well the standards were met and if not, identify reasons for this.

Stage 4: **Making Improvements:** Present the results to the relevant multidisciplinary teams in your organisation. Develop, agree and implement an action plan to bring actual practice closer to the standard.

Stage 5: **Sustaining Improvements:** After time for the intervention to take effect, collect new data and determine the impact. Then comparing again with the standard and establish if there was an improvement in practice (9, 10, 13, 22, 29–32)

Example of an audit cycle

1. Identifying a problem, e.g., long queue at discharge counter of the organisation

2. Defining standards/criteria, e.g., waiting time for 95% discharges should be less than an hour.

3. Collect data, e.g., record waiting hours, more time-consuming processes, personnel shortages.

4. Analysis, e.g. find out areas for improvement.

This framework looks similar to quality improvement (QI) process but QI process are shorter and follow the plan, do, study, act (PDSA) framework and aim to bring a holistic improvement in patient satisfaction (3, 6, 30).

Topics in an Audit: The following questions can be used as a guide to decide and prioritise a topic for auditing:

- Is there any evidence of resource wastage or risky practices?
- Is there any evidence of a serious quality issues; for example, poor feedback from beneficiaries?
- Are standardised guidelines available to compare the problem in question?
- Is there a possible and sustainable solution to the problem?
- Is the problem rampant and your solution can open newer avenues for policy making?
- Is the problem high on the priority list of your organisation? (3, 9, 29, 33)

Criteria: A definable measurable item of healthcare that describes quality and can be used to assess it. In an audit, the quality level of the outcome as well as the factors that effect on the service delivery becomes the criteria by which judgments are made. Each item together with the characteristics being looked at is a criterion. e.g., patients with glaucoma who have had their intra-occular pressure checked within the last 3 months. Criteria should be evidence-based wherever possible.

Criteria can be classified into those concerned with:

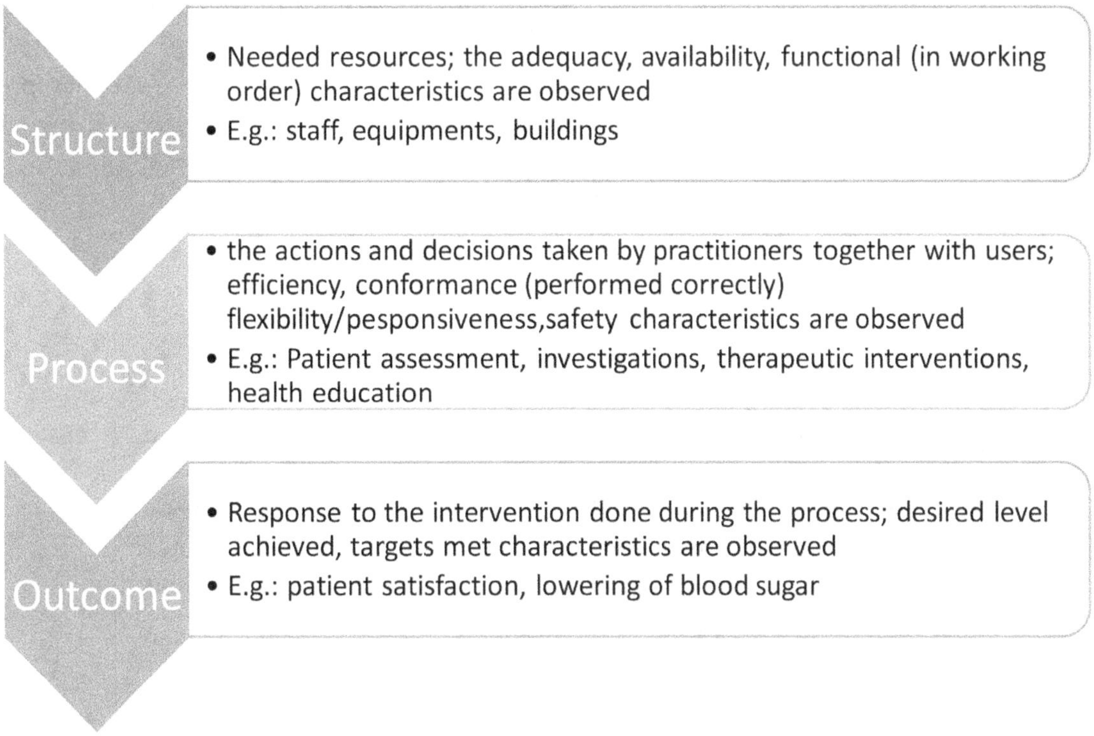

Structure
- Needed resources; the adequacy, availability, functional (in working order) characteristics are observed
- E.g.: staff, equipments, buildings

Process
- the actions and decisions taken by practitioners together with users; efficiency, conformance (performed correctly) flexibility/pesponsiveness,safety characteristics are observed
- E.g.: Patient assessment, investigations, therapeutic interventions, health education

Outcome
- Response to the intervention done during the process; desired level achieved, targets met characteristics are observed
- E.g.: patient satisfaction, lowering of blood sugar

Figure 2: Classification of Criteria

These criteria can be explicit or implicit.

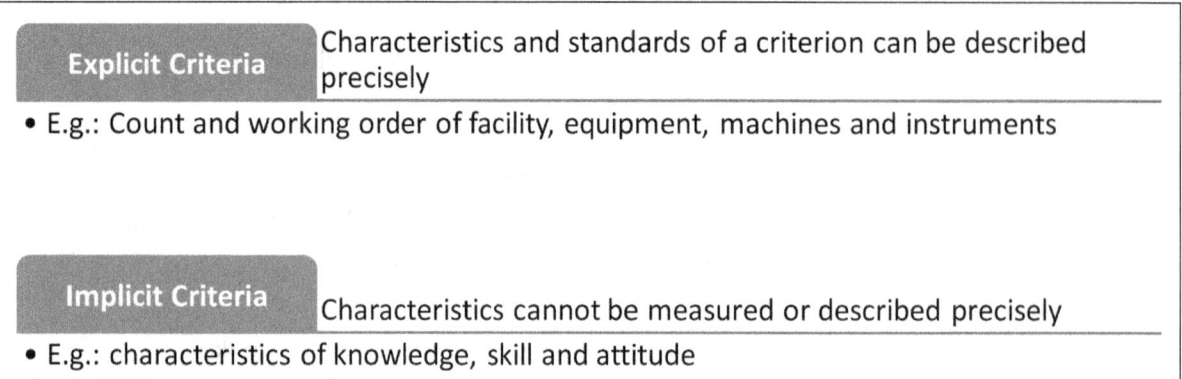

Figure 3: Explicit and Implicit Criteria

Standards: Standards describe the level of care desired or the value to be achieved for any particular characteristic. These standards may be set by the audit team itself or universally accepted standards can be used. For example, percentage of complication-free surgical cases can be set at 80 per cent, percentage of highly satisfied patients may be set at 90 per cent (2, 29, 32).

Audit Project Teams

An audit project team customised according to the specific audit project is formed keeping in mind to include members from all pertinent groups so as to meet the complete skill set requirement for a successful audit. For example, clinical service representatives, clinicians, nursing staff, infection control team, patient representatives and audit staff are usually included in audit project teams.

For a successful audit, all project team members should have:

- A basic understanding and training in clinical audit before starting the cycle
- An understanding of and commitment to the plans and objectives of the project
- An understanding of expectations from the audit team and the audit cycle

Role of Hospital Administration in Medical Audit/Quality Assurance

- Facilitation of good working environment, facilities and resources to conduct the audit
- Motivation and appraisal to health care professionals for performance of their duties
- Patient satisfaction surveys and exit interviews to unearth areas for improvement.
- Quick and satisfactory grievance redressal
- Media coverage
- Facilitate framing and implementation of objectives & policies after the audit (17).

Disseminating an Audit Report

Timely dissemination of a comprehensible and accessible audit report is more impactful in bringing about a change in practice and in turn formation of new national policies. It is also important to note the intended audience of the audit, a decade old arsenic contamination audit of Bangladesh in a small sample size will find little importance in Uttarakhand, India. Hence, timely revision of the audit with changes in patient load, time period and area is important for the audit to stay in relevance with evolving policies.

Changing Clinical Practice

With changes in policies post audit, changing clinical practice is a tedious task. Policy changes at national level and its dissemination to lower levels can take years as it takes several cycles of refining, resetting and achieving standards to improve standards of patient care. An organisation with history of impeccable infrastructure, good work culture, focus on quality improvement, regular audit cycles, motivated team members and a high national and international visibility is more likely to expedite the process. A regular audit cycle that sets standards, measures, reflects, implement changes, review standards and repeats the whole cycle is more likely to maximise its impact on current practices in patient care. (22, 32).

Summary

Audits are handy tools for quality improvement used to identify hiccups in patient care and provide sustainable solutions. They include identifying the problem, setting defining criteria and standards for the problem and initiating an audit cycle, which is maintained by an audit team. The essential steps include: planning for audit, standard/criteria selection, data collection and measuring performance, making improvements, sustaining improvements. The results of the cycle essentially deal with the outcome and should be disseminated timely to the relevant audience to make an impact on current medical practices and to influence national policies (10).

Further Reading:

- Clare Mayo Gill Harvey. *The Clinical Audit Book*,1st ed. Elsevier,
- Brian W. Kozic. *The Healthcare Auditor's Handbook*. HCPro, Inc.
- Robin Burgess, and John Moorhead. *New Principles of Best Practice in Clinical Audit*, 1st ed. CRC Press, 2011.
- Simon P Frostick, Philip J Radford, and W Angus Wallace. *Medical Audit: Rationale and Practicalities*. Cambridge University Press, 2009.

References

1. Cambridge English Dictionary. Audit [Internet]. Cambridge English Dictionary. [cited 2021 Feb 9]. Available from: https://dictionary.cambridge.org/dictionary/english/audit

2. P Esposito. 'Clinical Audit, A Valuable Tool to Improve Quality of Care: General Methodology and Applications in Nephrology'. *World J Nephrol* [Internet]. 2014 [cited 2021 Feb 9];3(4):249. Available from: /pmc/articles/PMC4220358/

3. I Kakande. 'Clinical and Medical Audit: What it is and What to do'. East Cent African J Surg [Internet], 8(1). 2003 [cited 10 February 2021]. Available from: https://www.ajol.info/index.php/ecajs/article/view/136764

4. PC Modayil, RK Panchikkeel, and N Alex. 'Audit in Clinical Practice'. *Indian J Otolaryngol Head Neck Surg* [Internet], 61(2): pp 109–11. June 2009 [cited 21 February 2021]. Available from: www.nice.org.uk

5. A Soliman. 'Principles of Methodological Design of Clinical Audit'. *Arch Med* [Internet]. 22 March 2018 [cited 8 February 2021]; 10(2). Available from: http://www.imedpub.com/

6. R Juyal, and V Vallabh.' Quality in Health Care'. In: AM Kadri, ed. *IAPSM Textbook of Community Medicine* [Internet]. 1st ed, p 1018–25. New Delhi: Jaypee Publishers, 2019 [cited 21 February 2021].

7. C Fawkes, AP Moore, C Peers, B McIlwraith, and K Chorley. 'A Brief Introduction to Clinical Audit' [Internet]. London; 2000 [cited 9 February 2021]. Available from: www.gp-training.net

8. LAB Camacho, and HR Rubin. 'Reliability of Medical Audit in Quality Assessment of Medical Care'. *Cad Saude Publica*, 12(suppl 2): pp S85–93 [Internet]. 1996 [cited 8 February 2021].

9. UBHT Clinical Audit Central Office. 'How to Do a Clinical Audit: A Brief Guide [Internet], 3rd ed. UBHT Clinical Audit Central Office, ed, Vol 2. Bristol: National Health Services, pp 1–5; 2007 [cited 9 February 2021]. Available from: www.nice.org.uk/pdf/BestPracticeClinicalAudit.pdf

10. JR Colvin, and CJ Peden, ed. 'Raising the Standard: A Compendium of Audit Recipes' [Internet]. 3rd ed. *London: The Royal College of Anaesthetists*; 2012 [cited 9 February 2021]. Available from: www.rcoa.ac.uk

11. DA Roberts. "'Working for Patients' the 1989 White Paper on the Health Service: An Over-Review and Commentary". *Teach Public Adm* [Internet], 9(1): pp 33–40. 31 March 1989 [cited 21 February 2021]. Available from: http://journals.sagepub.com/doi/10.1177/014473948900900103

12. MM Singh, and R Devi. 'Clinical Audit: More of a Dream Than a Reality in India'. *BMJ* [Internet]. 3 April 2014 [cited 8 February 2021]; 348. Available from: https://www.bmj.com/content/348/bmj.g2514

13. AT Hexter. 'How to Conduct a Clinical Audit: A Guide for Medical Students'. Manchester; 2013.

14. CD Shaw, and DW Costain. 'Guidelines for Medical Audit: Seven Principles'. *Br Med J* [Internet], 299 (6697): pp 498–99. 19 August 1989 [cited 8 February 2021]. Available from: http://www.bmj.com/

15. A Shennan, A Briley. 'Clinical Research Methodology'. *Basic Science in Obstetrics and Gynaecology* [Internet], pp 305–16. Elsevier, 2010 [cited 8 February 2021]. Available from: https://linkinghub.elsevier.com/retrieve/pii/B9780443102813000191

16. P Thirumalaikolundusubramanian, M Ramachandran, and S Senthilkumaran. 'Ethics, Legality, and Education in the Practice of Cardiology'. *Heart and Toxins,* pp 595–623. Elsevier Inc, 2015.

17. Y Sharma, and P Mahajan. 'Role of Medical Audit in Health Care Evaluation'. *JK Sci J Med Educ Res,* 1(4): pp 193–96. December 1999.

18. CM McKee, M Lauglo, and L Lessof. 'Medical Audit: A Review'. *J R Soc Med,* 82: pp 474–78 [Internet]. August 1989 [cited 8 February 2021]. Available from: https://www.ncbi.nlm.nih.gov/pmc/articles/PMC1292253/pdf/jrsocmed00147-0028.pdf

19. D Sellu. 'Time to Audit Audit'. *BMJ,* 312(7023): p 128 [Internet]. 13 January 1996 [cited 22 February 2021]. Available from: https://www.bmj.com/content/312/7023/128.2

20. U Perumal, M Rajivlochan, and S Nundy. 'The Importance of Clinical Audit in India'. *Curr Med Res Pract,* 10 (3): pp 110–15.. 1 May 2020.

21. KB O'Reilly. '13 Reasons Your Practice Should Have a Medical Record Audit [Internet]. *American Medical Association.* [cited 9 February 2021]. Available from: https://www.ama-assn.org/practice-management/cpt/13-reasons-your-practice-should-have-medical-record-audit

22. C Paton, and TRE Barnes. 'Undertaking Clinical Audit, with Reference to a Prescribing Observatory for Mental Health Audit of Lithium Monitoring'. *Psychiatr Bull,* 38(3): pp 128–31 [Internet]. June 2014 [cited 9 February 2021]. Available from: /pmc/articles/PMC4115378/

23. SK Patnaik, MM Singh, and B Sridhar. 'Medical Audit of Documentation of Inpatient Medical Record in a Multispecialty Hospital in India'. *Int J Res Found Hosp Healthc Adm,* 5(2): pp 77–83. December 2017.

24. SW Mercer, K Sevar, and TD Sadutshan. 'Using Clinical Audit to Improve the Quality of Obstetric Care at the Tibetan Delek Hospital in North India: A Longitudinal Study'. *Reprod Health,* 7; 3:4–4. June 2006.

25. S Chaturvedi, P Sinha, P Chandra, and G Desai. 'Improving Quality of Prescriptions with Clinical Audit'. *Indian J Med Sci,* 62 (11): pp 461–64. 1 November 2008.

26. M Kameswaran, S Raghunandhan, K Natarajan, and N Basheeth. 'Clinical Audit of Outcomes in Cochlear Implantation an Indian Experience'. *Indian J Otolaryngol Head Neck Surg,* 58 (1): pp 69–73. January 2006.

27. Faculty of Public Health. 'Quality Improvement Activity' [Internet]. 2021 [cited 9 February 2021. Available from: https://www.fph.org.uk/professional-development/revalidation/how-to-prepare-for-your -revalidation/quality-improvement-activity/

28. National Health Agency, Ayushman Bharat Pradhan Mantri Jan Arogya Yojana. Fraud Investigation and Medical Audit Manual. December 2018.

29. Radcliffe Medical Press. 'Principles for Best Practice in Clinical Audit' [Internet]. Abingdon; 2002 [cited 9 February 2021]. Available from: www.radcliffe-oxford.com

30. C Limb, A Fowler, B Gundogan, K Koshy, and R Agha. 'How to Conduct a Clinical Audit and Quality Improvement Project'. *Int J Surg Oncol,* 2(6): pp e24–e24 [Internet]. July 2017 [cited 9 February 2021]. Available from: /pmc/articles/PMC5673151/

31. Faculty of Public Health Medicine. 'Clinical Audit/Quality Improvement Projects Guidance For Professional Competence Scheme' [Internet]. December 2012 [cited 9 February 2021]. Available from: https://rcpi-live-cdn.s3.amazonaws.com/wp-content/uploads/2016/01/PCS-FPHM-Audit_Quality-Guide.pdf

32. G Copeland. 'A Practical Handbook for Clinical Audit' [Internet]. National Health Services, ed, pp 1–49. Contact Details Clinical Governance Support Team 1st Floor, St John's House 30 East Street Leicester: Clinical Governance Support Team; 2005 [cited 9 February 2021].

33. T Jones, and S Cawthorn. 'What is Clinical Audit?' Hayward Medical Communications [Internet]. 2002 [cited 22 February 2021]; Available from:

34. J Grimshaw, I Shirran, R Thomas, G Mowatt, C Fraser, L Bero, et al. 'Changing Provider Behavior: An Overview of Systematic Reviews of Interventions. *Med Care,* 39 (8): pp 112–45 [Internet]. 2001 Aug [cited 22 February 2021]. Available from: https://pubmed.ncbi.nlm.nih.gov/11583120/

CHAPTER 11

Electronic Medical Records

Dr. Indranil Chakrabarti

Additional Professor, Department of Pathology

AIIMS Kalyani, West Bengal

Record keeping and documentation of patients' medical history form a very important component of patient health care. With the improvement of healthcare system and reduction of acute diseases, more and more patients are now suffering from various chronic illnesses.

They often have a long history of medical and surgical consultations which becomes very relevant in their subsequent treatment decisions.

Traditionally, all the details of the patient were being stored manually in a paper-based system also known as medical charts. However, besides being labor intensive and time consuming, there were problems regarding security of data, consumption of space and also the risk of information being misplaced or lost.

With the advent of computers, these records gradually were started to be stored in computers as a single file of the hospital record keeping section in the name of the patient. However, it was gradually felt that not only is the storage of data important, but the ease of access and retrieval should also be kept in mind.

With the advancement of Information and Communication Technologies (ICTs), the Medical Informatics System(MIS) has come up with several solutions to these problems. The Electronic Medical Records (EMR) is one such solution which can act as a repository of all patient information in the form of digital documents. It incorporates the medical, surgical and personal history of patients including allergies, drug history, summary of all the patients' visits, observations, radiology and laboratory investigations and treatment that has been rendered in the treating institution.[1]The data can be stored on-premise or in cloud-based systems and can subsequently be accessed by authorized personnel.

In general, health care providers of our country are very reluctant to maintain patient records and even in many advanced set-ups, the patient file is limited to a paper or plastic folder loaded with prescriptions, laboratory reports and data sheets of previous visits of the patient to the hospital. But now, the EMR provides a much smarter and secure solution of data handling aimed at maintaining a complete and comprehensivepatient profile.

Its advantages can thus be enumerated as the following:[1,2]

    i. Less expensive

    ii. Less time consuming for the health care providers who can do away with much paperwork

    iii. Reduction in the likelihood of error in health care as all previous medical, surgical history available easily

    iv. Avoidance of mistakes arising from illegible handwriting or using confusing acronyms resulting in errors in patient names, medications, diagnosis or even treatment provided

    v. Reduction of costs due to avoidance of duplication of tests and procedures

    vi. Less chance of loss or misplacement

    vii. Less consumption of space

    viii. Can be preserved for longer periods

    ix. Security of access to patient records can be ensured by allowing access only to authorized personnel

    x. Ready accessibility of important highlights of the patient

    xi. Can even be remotely accessed if the data is stored in cloud-based applications

    xii. Helpful for analysis and further research activities as stored in a digital format

    xiii. Records can be utilized for education, regulation, surveillance and quality assurance.

    xiv. Suitable for health care providers in speciality clinics

    xv. Less rejection of health insurance claims

    xvi. Helpful in medicolegal suits

However, such digitalization of medical records also faces certain challenges, the greatest being adapting to the change by sceptical users and those with limited IT skills. The barriers, thus, can be listed as follows:

    i. Lack of intent to adapt to a new technology

    ii. Lack of awareness about the advantages of digitalization

    iii. Concern about increased cost as the initial investment

    iv. Dedicated staff for maintenance of records and availability of trained manpower

    v. Transferring the paper-based records to electronic format

    vi. Concern regarding the security, confidentiality and privacy of patient information

    vii. Lack of certification

With the advancement of the Electronic healthcare records (ECHR) system, there has been increasing need for more completeness and accessibility of the patient data. While EMR can be looked upon as a digitalized medical record of a patient available at one organization, the concept has now been extended to the evolution of a system to encompass the entire health record of the patient from all the treating institutes into one all-encompassing data format which is known as Electronic Health Record or EHR. EHR has been defined as digitally stored healthcare information about an individual's lifetime with the purpose ofsupporting continuity of care, education and research, and ensuring confidentiality at alltimes.[3]This allows of sharing of patient data so that the treating physician can have access to all the previous health records of the patient in previous institutions as well as allowing him/her a better understanding of the patient condition and thus facilitating better management. The major advantages of EHR over EMR are that the information can be shared electronically between the healthcare providers and that it is certifiable. The EHR software programs not only ensure smarter healthcare delivery but they also reduce staff workload and reduce the chance of errors.

This software can also be integrated with office management software to build a Patient management (PM) software which can ensure setting appointments and billing as well.

While EHR is maintained by organization(s), there has also been emergence of a patient health care record system known as Personal health record or PHR.

PHR has been defined as an electronic, universally available, lifelong resource of health related information maintained and owned by the individual patient.[4] It includes information obtained from healthcare providers as well as the patient himself/herself. It ensures the privacy and safety of the information as only the individual determines the right to access.

Standardisation of such record keeping and the feasibility of implementation of various e-health initiatives remain challenging but as the use of the ECHR is more than the abuse, it is being increasingly adapted in most of the developed countries of Europe and United States of America. Some of the biggest corporate hospitals and academic institutes of India are also using the digitalized patient records with the aim of improving quality, efficacy and safety of patients with better health outcomes. With artificial intelligence and e-prescribing making inroads in day to day practice it seems inevitable that all healthcare personnel have to adapt to these modern technologies better sooner than later.

References

1. M R Mane, D.R. Kulkarni(2012): A Review: Electronic Medical Records (EMR) System for Clinical Data Storage at health centers. Available at: https://www.semanticscholar.org/paper/A-Review-%3A-Electronic-Medical-Records-(-EMR-)-for-Mane-Kulkarni/82f4cdf02af73ac4e78448e89e34111696f2945d
   [Accessed on 18.03.2021]
2. A V Athavale, S P Zodpey(2010): Public health informatics in India: The potential and the challenges. Indian J Public Health vol. 4, pp. 131-136.
3. I. Iakovidis (1998) "Towards Personal Health Record: Current situation, obstacles and trends in implementation of Electronic Healthcare Records in Europe", International Journal of Medical Informatics vol. 52 no. 128, pp. 105 –117.
4. Peter J. Groen, Douglas Goldstein, Jaime Nasuti (2007): Personal Health Record (PHR) Systems: An Evolving Challenge to EHR Systems. Available at http://www.hoise.com/vmw/07/articles/vmw/LV-VM-08-07-26.html [Accessed on 21.03.2021]

CHAPTER 12

Accreditation, Benchmarking and Quality Control in Health Management

Dr Sanjeev Kumar

Associate Professor, Department of Community and Family Medicine

All India Institute of Medical Sciences Bhopal, Madhya Pradesh

EVOLUTION OF QUALITY CONTROL IN HEALTH MANAGEMENT

How has the quality control and quality assurance in health management evolved?

Access to universal healthcare need to go in tandem with quality of care. The need to constantly recognize, analyze and eliminate variations in indicators of healthcare provision has been long identified. Methods of quality control in healthcare were adopted from industrial quality science. The analogy of client satisfaction from business sector has been incorporated into patient satisfaction and improved outcomes of healthcare delivery.

Healthcare has slowly evolved from the provision of patronizing 'art' of prescribing to participatory, evidence-based and dynamic 'service'. During this journey, innovative concepts propounded by stalwarts such as Dr. W A Shewhart, W. Edwards Deming, Joseph Juran, Ernest Codman, Kaoru Ishikawa, Bill Smith, Masaaki Imai, Avedis Donabedian etc have shaped the current body of literature on quality management in healthcare. As early as 1854-56, Florence Nightingale demonstrated the effect of thoughtful observation in provision of healthcare and successfully instituted hygienic measures to decrease the mortality rates among soldiers during Crimean War. Shewhart introduced the concept of *"control charts"* and *Plan-Do-Study-Act* (PDSA) cycles. Deming popularized the PDSA cycle in Japan. This subsequently led to the quality revolution in the country's industrial sector and motivated many others such as Ishikawa to dwell upon quality concepts to come up with famed *'Fishbone diagrams'* of quality assurance. Ernest Codman is credited with strengthening the accreditation of hospitals through *Joint Commission on Accreditation of Hospitals* in USA as early as 1950s which was probably the first such impartial organization. Initial impetus of quality improvement had been to obtain cost-effectiveness in production and obtain greater gains. Subsequently, it has included processes too. Donabedian, considered as the father of healthcare quality, introduced the classification of quality indicators into structure, process and outcome.

Quality control slowly either metamorphosed or included other dimensions of quality and got to be known by terminologies such as quality assurance, quality management, continuous quality management, total quality management etc. Continuous quality improvement (CQI) and Total Quality Management (TQM) were ushered in after techniques of identifying and reducing deviations in processes were innovated and tested by pioneers such as Juran's *quality trilogy*, Bill Smith's *Six Sigma* in Motorola and Toyota's *Kaizen methods*.

In 1985, accreditation agencies of various countries collaborated to form ISQua (International Society for Quality in Healthcare) in order to bring about harmonization in the process of quality management and accreditation.

There are certain terms and concept which would constantly be mentioned in this chapter. These need to be referred again and again. You should be familiar with these terms and concepts first. Since these have been listed at one place, it should be easier for you to refer this section whenever required.

Terms	Explanation
Quality	Quality is the degree to which a service conforms to accepted standards and expectations of consumer. In healthcare delivery, patient and their family members are the "consumers". While "service" can be consultation with a doctor or nurse, laboratory procedure (tests on samples of blood/urine/tissue), imaging (X-ray, Ultrasonography, CT Scan), allied processes (food, drinking water, toilet facilities, linen etc).
Standard	Standard is a predefined parameter against which values determined by observing or measuring a healthcare-related variable is compared. Standards are decided by statutory agencies or other autonomous organizations. Parameters considered as standards are agreed upon by all the concerned stakeholders. Standards are usually a minimum set of criteria of performance. For example, every hospital must display a patient charter of rights. NABH defines standards as a statement of expectations that defines the structures and processes that must be substantially in place in an organization to enhance the quality of care.
Indicator	Indicator is a specific, observable or measurable characteristic used to objectively designate the status or performance of a variable. Indicators of healthcare may belong to input, process, output, outcome, or impact. Indicators are often used in supervision, monitoring and evaluation in healthcare. For example, proportion of vacant positions of ANM is an input indicator, while number of trainings on biomedical waste management is a process indicator. Proportion of satisfied patients in an outpatient setting is outcome indicator. Mortality rates are impact indicators. NABH defines indicator as a statistical measure of the performance of functions, systems or processes over time.
Benchmark	Benchmark is a point of reference against which something can be compared with. Benchmarks are like standards but are used when an organization wishes to improve its quality of care. For example, a newly established hospital may choose to provide digital X-rays to at least 50% of its patients at the same rate within next 6 months as compared to currently no such facility being available.
Quality control	This usually is limited to efforts taken by facilities or organization to simply comply with predefined measurable minimum standards. Quality control aims at *preventing* healthcare-associated errors. For example, hospitals need to get registered with Central Pollution Control Board (CPCB) and segregate sharp waste into white translucent puncture-proof dustbins to prevent needlestick injuries among staff, patients and waste-handlers.

Terms	Explanation
Quality assurance	Quality assurance is focused on *finding and correcting* the healthcare-associated errors. It involves planned and systematic approach to monitor, assess and improve quality on a continuous basis within the existing resources. For example, National Tuberculosis Elimination Programme has a quality assurance system known as EQUAS (External Quality Assessment System). This system identifies if any laboratory technician is making consistent errors in slide preparation or reporting and need to be trained. Quality assurance can be carried out by designated quality assurance personnel or someone from the department itself. In the example on EQUAS, Senior TB Laboratory Supervisor (STLS) performs quality assurance.
Quality improvement	It aims at *raising* the quality of health services. It identifies areas of problems in the health system, conducts root-cause analysis, develops step-wise solutions and tests such solutions. For example, a healthcare wanting to obtain ISO certification may seek professional help in identifying problems areas in its crowd management to improve client satisfaction. Quality improvement goes a notch beyond quality assurance.
Total Quality Management (TQM)	Total quality management aims to *improve* process in such a manner that at an acceptable cost, functional health of patients is improved, and they are satisfied with the process of care as well. The decision makers in the hospital or programme managers need to first accept that they believe in utility of TQM as one of the means to achieve health-related goals. But to be a proponent of TQM, the goals should not be numerical and enforced work-standards should be done away with. Personnel management strategy should change with objective of elimination of harmful variations in structure, process and outcome of the hospital or the programme. A culture of continuous training needs to be incorporated.
Benchmarking	In benchmarking, performance of a healthcare facility or programme is compared with the best-performing facility or programme. In this approach, current indicators are compared with a known standard belonging to leaders in industry or service. For example, an eye hospital may seek to obtain ISO certification on using the most-advanced laser technique for corneal surgery because the most famous hospital of the city has that certificate.
Accreditation	It is process of assessment of a healthcare organization to pre-determined and published standards. It is usually voluntary and ongoing process. By this process, an authoritative body formally recognizes the competence of the organization in providing services belonging to specified standards. Accreditation is usually performed by an independent third-party organization. For example, in India National Accreditation Board of Hospitals and Healthcare Providers (NABH) does this. NABH defines accreditation as self-assessment and external peer-review process used by healthcare organizations to accurately assess their level of performance in relation to established standards and to implement ways to improve the healthcare system continuously.

Need, Means and Ends of Quality Control in Health Management

What is the need of quality control in health management?

A popular myth among healthcare managers is that adoption of quality control measures would increase cost of healthcare. Research has shown it to be otherwise. Investing in improving quality of healthcare reduces overall cost of care. Nearly 80% of Indians obtain ambulatory healthcare in India through private health system. Since holistic healthcare is one of the ends of health policy in India, various health programmes are run by both union and state governments. Resources are finite, while expectations of people and concerns of government are infinite. Hence, processes and interventions need to be periodically checked for cost-effectiveness. Often, hospitals and health programmes report numbers as parameters of success. For example, 'n' number of surgeries conducted in a year or 'k' number of patients consulted in a camp. But even the best programme should be considered only partially successful if all intended beneficiaries don't want to, or can't reach to, or can't afford to use it. Hence, during monitoring of the hospital services and healthcare programmes, quality becomes as important as quantity. It is not enough to only report about finishing a 'procedure' or immunizing a child or buying the product from the vendor quoting lowest price.

The success of automobile industry of Japan is a prime example. As compared to the assembly line of production of cars in Ford Motors, Japanese automobile manufacturers slowly introduced concepts of identifying the errors during driving and trying to minimize them. The resultant safety helped boost the confidence of buyers so much in Japanese cars that they slowly overtook Ford Motors as leading manufacturers. The concept of Six Sigma (i.e. reducing errors to less than six standard deviation) was one of the goals of these manufacturers. Loyally of customers in manufacturing sector can be compared with likelihood of having continuity-of-seeking healthcare in country like India where most of care is sought in form of cross- or split-referrals.

Standards may be led down by government or mutually agreed upon by the leaders of the sector or based on the expectations and value-judgement by clients (ie patients/care-seekers). Quality assurance is the ongoing development of criteria and standards on provision of quality services/products and tracking of these services/products through indicators.

How can quality control be achieved in a hospital or health programme?

To achieve quality control, actual performance of healthcare system (hospitals or health programmes) is measured and compared with standards or benchmarks to identify shortcoming. Subsequently action need to be taken by decision makers to solve these shortcomings. Finally, an ongoing monitoring system need to be developed to check whether the quality control intervention has succeeded. The PDSA or PDCA cycle can be an easy mnemonic for this process (figure 1). During "Plan" stage, we need to identify what change is required or what needs to be improved. During "Do" stage, desired change or improvement is implemented. During "Study", we measure and analyse the process or outcome emanating from the implemented change or improvement. At last, during "Act" phase, we observe whether we achieved what we aspired during "Plan" stage. In the PDCA cycle, the "Check" stage uses checklists to objectively check changes or improvements.

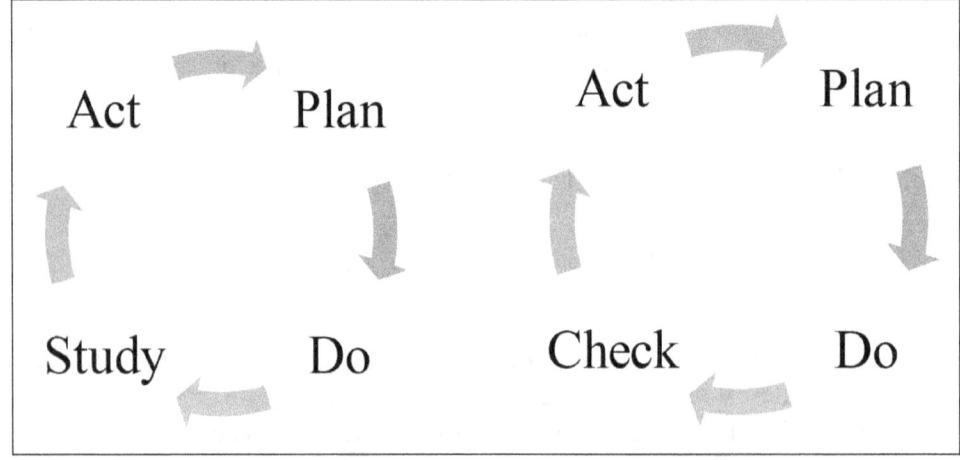

Figure 1: PDSA & PDCA Cycles

Continuous quality improvement (CQI) has been another paradigm in quality control in healthcare. CQI team in hospitals often starts problem identification through techniques of brainstorming, flowcharting, matrix or fishbone (Ishikawa) diagrams. Problem areas can be identified through client flow analysis, tally sheets, graphical visualization aids (bar charts, histograms, stratification, Scatter or control/Shewhart chart), pareto analysis etc. Use of standards such as ISO 9000 series can be a way of CQI to achieve TQM. For health programmes, evaluation techniques such as logical framework, CFIR (Consolidated Framework for Implementation Research) etc can be adopted or adapted.

Quality of healthcare in hospitals involves both technical care (i.e. diagnostic and therapeutic procedures) and art of care (i.e. behavariour of providers). The usual annual reports of hospitals and health programme in India usually mention outputs of the technical care in form of frequencies and percentages. Quality of healthcare has recently received impetus in India as exemplified first through launch of NABH, IPHS and NQAS standards, then in form of initiatives like Kayakalp and Mera Aspatal for public health facilities.

Dimensions of Quality

Assessment of quality requires identification of its dimensions. Many attempts have been made to classify dimensions of quality. In its simplest form, quality is classified into two dimensions conforming to either specifications or customer requirements reflecting the perspectives of expert view and customer. For conformance to specifications, measurements are obtained over time and compared with either average performance of the organization itself (eg by using Control Charts) or with a predefined indicator (standard or benchmark). World Health Organization (WHO) advocates quality assessment across six dimensions of being effective, efficient, accessible, acceptable (patient-centered), equitable and safe. Table 1 compares the dimensions of quality considered by some acclaimed organizations.

Table 1: Dimensions of quality identified by agencies

AHRQ	IOM	WHO	JCAHO
Effective	Effective	Effective	Effectiveness
Efficient	Efficient	Efficient	Efficiency
Equitable	Equitable	Equitable	Availability
Patient-centered	Patient-centered	Acceptable/patient-centred	Respect & caring
Safe	Safe	Safe	Safety
Timely	Timely	Accessible	Timeliness
			Appropriateness
			Continuity
			Efficacy

Many other expert-developed quality of care assessment tools also mention dimensions of quality. Patient satisfaction tools are often developed around certain dimensions. For example, Gavin identified 8 dimensions. Lindsay & Evans also mentioned 8 separate dimensions. Scales like Patient Satisfaction Questionnaire (PSQ) 18, SERVQUAL, KQCAH etc use overlapping as well as unique dimensions. PSQ-18 measure indicators related to the physical environment like accessibility of the hospital, convenience or location of the health facility and the presence of basic amenities.

Standards are developed to measure quality in the agreed dimensions. Standards should be valid, reliable, sensitive and specific. Process standards are often more desirable in quality control as compared to outcome standards. Standards can be checked either through self-assessment or during inspection or through accreditation. To track the implementation of quality control, indicators must be developed. An indicator is considered as a tool which helps in guiding data collection. It is measurable, but are different from standard. Some indicators can be number of services available, specialization of doctors, their performance in specific diseases, poor practice leading to disciplinary action, adverse events, hospital mortality etc. Table 2 depicts examples of indicators across the domains of structure, process and outcomes.

Table 2: Examples of indicators across domains of structure, process and outcome

Structure (or Input) Indicators	Process Indicators	Outcome indicators
❖ physical facility – space, number of beds, number of OTs, types of OTs, proximity to modes of transport etc ❖ interdepartmental relationship of functional units (eg presence of committee and board such as condemnation committee or tumour board etc) ❖ human resources – qualification, expertise & experience, job description, job content, job analysis at each position, knowledge & skill required, recruitment policy, human resource development policy, trainings (orientation/ongoing), defined & written duty/responsibilities of staff, supervision policy & guidelines etc ❖ staffing norms, selection criteria, selection process ❖ equipment with appropriate technology, purchase committee, purchase system, installation & maintenance programme, periodic validation, repair facilities, operation manuals, training ❖ materials (medicines, surgical items, dietary supplies etc) - demand assessment, specifications, drug formulary, drug selection committee, purchase committees, purchasing system, procedures on receipt/inspection//storage/issue, store management etc	❖ medical care ❖ nursing care ❖ supportive & utility care ❖ process evaluation through medical/nursing audit or peer review or death review or tissue review, medical records committee, utilization committee, hospital infection control committee, patient care committee, grievance committee etc	❖ average length of stay ❖ complications rate ❖ readmission rate ❖ hospital infection rates ❖ death rates ❖ patient satisfaction ❖ hospital acquired infection rate ❖ referral rate

Steps of Quality Management in Healthcare

Health management consists of planning, implementation and monitoring. Quality control in healthcare essentially follow similar process. Here planning would consist of situational analysis followed by stakeholder engagement to decide on areas of improvement, standards and indicators etc. As part of implementation of quality control and assurance, data is collected, collated, analyzed and shared with decision makers in the organization to take correcting action. Monitoring of quality can be done through analysis of management information system (MIS), patient satisfaction surveys and feedback, or external survey. Figure 2 demonstrates schematics for steps of quality control in a hospital.

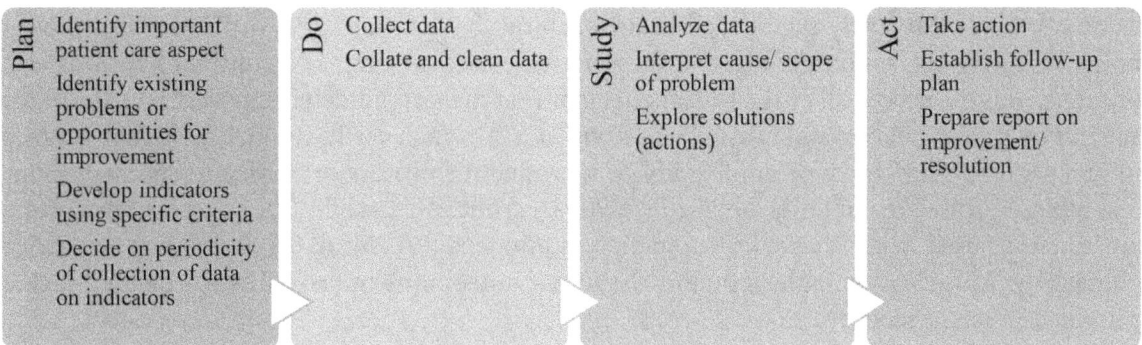

Figure 2: Steps of quality control in a hospital

During action stage, staff engagement is one of the key steps in quality control, assurance and improvement. Health managers can use behaviour theories such as 'diffusion of innovation' or 'risk communication' to identify early adopters of change, resisters and fence-sitters. Champions of change to achieve the improved quality should be identified as they can guide and motivate the 'silent boosters' (positive fence-sitters). By using influence-interest grid, managers should list and classify the 'blockers' (i.e. the active resisters who are usually a few in numbers), and identify those who can have enough influence on the 'avoiders' (negative fence-sitters who usually are in larger numbers) to affect the process of change towards better quality. Afterwards, by seeking help of influential champions, the negative campaigns by the 'blockers' should be fended off.

For quality assurance, either benchmarks can be identified by health managers or accreditation can be sought from appropriate agencies (eg NABH or NABL in India, JCI in USA etc). Major steps of quality assurance are definition, measurement and evaluation.

Goals of Quality Control in Healthcare Management

The overall goal of quality management in healthcare system is to achieve best-possible health outcomes in the patients with the limited resources. These outcomes can be expressed in form of summary measures which can be captured as indicators. The benchmarks and standards which themselves are indicators or measures agreed upon as local (or national) voluntary (or necessary) targets may serve as the next level of goals of quality. Apart from outcomes, the focus of quality management in healthcare has included the process of healthcare too. Hence, the goals of quality should be to improve process of care, increase and sustain patient satisfaction, improve functional health of patients and reduce costs.

Quality management may achieve one of the following ends –

(A) Self-assessment: Here standards may have either been set by the organization itself or by an outside agency or government. It is not legally binding to conduct self-assessment. Self-assessment may be conducted either for the entire hospital or for individual department. Health programme may also undergo self-assessment by senior managers in form of periodic monitoring and supervision. Medical audit which was started in 1950s in USA is a popular example of self-assessment. SWOT (Strength, Weakness, Opportunity, Threat) or SWOC (Challenge in place of Threat of SWOT) analysis and Force-Field analysis are other popular methods of self-assessment which can be applicable to both health facilities and health programmes. Example of self-assessment using standards set by other agency is the internal assessment phase under Kayakalp guidelines of government of India.

(B) Inspection and licensure: For inspection, standards are set by authorities such as union/central or state governments, or professional bodies (eg National Medical Commission, Central Pollution Control Bureau, FSSAI, CAG etc). These standards are usually in form of some legislation (eg PCPNDT Act 1994, Clinical Establishment Act 2010, Biomedical Waste Management Rules 2018, Factory's Act 1948, Environmental Protection Act etc). All newly established health facilities have to undergo inspection and showcase their 'compliance' to the set standards. Most of these activities are ongoing and continues periodically.

(C) Certification: It is the process of evaluation and recognition to meet pre-determined criteria. Certification may or may not be legally binding and is usually not ongoing. Through certification, a written assurance is given by an independent third-party on conformity of a product or process or service to specified requirements. For example, hospitals voluntarily obtain ISO 9001 certification, while BIS certification is necessary for certain materials used in healthcare (eg room air conditioners, PVC insulated heavy duty electric cables).

(D) Benchmarking: This is an example of quality assurance and quality improvement as defined earlier. Details are provided in next section.

(E) Accreditation: This is an example of quality assurance and quality improvement as defined earlier. Details are provided in next section.

Benchmarking and Accreditation in healthcare

What is benchmarking in healthcare?

As defined earlier, benchmarking is the process of comparing performance of a hospital or a health programme to that of the best existing examples. It is a component of TQM. Therefore, it must be a team process. Four types of benchmarking have been identified (see figure 2).

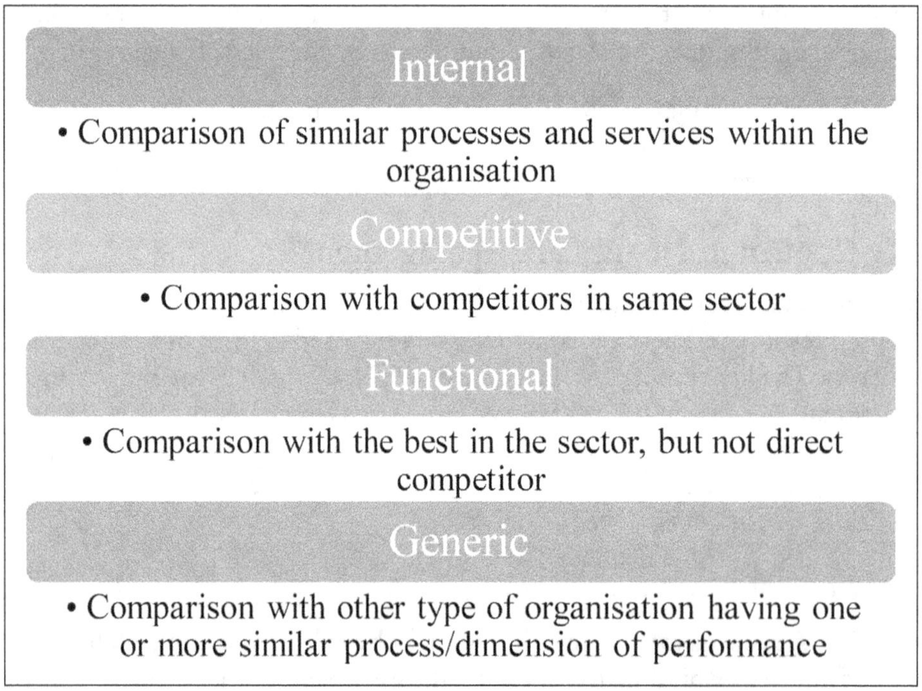

Internal
- Comparison of similar processes and services within the organisation

Competitive
- Comparison with competitors in same sector

Functional
- Comparison with the best in the sector, but not direct competitor

Generic
- Comparison with other type of organisation having one or more similar process/dimension of performance

Figure 2: Types of Benchmarking

What is accreditation in healthcare?

As defined earlier, accreditation can be considered as attestation by impartial experts on the competency to carry out specific tasks under pre-identified activities or services being provided by a health facility or organization. Various steps of accreditation include consultation with all stakeholders to decide on standards to be used, measuring current level of compliance with the standards, changes in processes to fill the gaps in compliance, and seeking assessment by accreditation agency. Accreditation can be obtained for the whole organization, a department, a unit or even a process. For example, internationally agreed standards for accreditation of laboratories are provided under ISO 15189 guidelines which is based on ISO/IEC standard 17025.

ISO 9000 was first published in 1987 by the International Organization for Standardization, a specialized international independent agency composed of national standard bodies of more than 160 countries. The standards were revised in 2000, 2008 and 2015. Healthcare related ISO standards are called ISO 9000 and ISO 9001.

Quality Management in Healthcare in India

How quality management in healthcare has evolved in India?

As pointed out earlier, global acceptance of quality in healthcare was imbibed from its success in domains of manufacturing, military and business management. Similarly in India too, formal interest in quality management emanated from need to improve manufactured products to compete in global markets. Following economic liberalization in India after 1991, the embargo on foreign-made goods was lifted. Indian manufacturers felt the heat of competition with other global manufacturers. The leading associations in business and manufacturing led to the formation of World Trade Organization (WTO) in 1995 as a quality yardstick agency. Quality Council of India (QCI) was set-up in 1997. Apart from quality monitoring of various sectors, healthcare quality became part of QCI.

How can benchmarking and accreditation in healthcare be obtained in India?

In India, private healthcare facilities and organization can voluntarily seek accreditation from various independent agencies such as NABH, NABL, ISO, JCI etc depending upon the services being rendered and spectrum of clientele. Public healthcare facilities can also use the standards laid down under IPHS (Indian Public Health Standards) and NQAS (National Quality Assurance Standards). NQAS standards are still not available for PHCs, HWCs (Health & Wellness Centres) and Subcentres. National Accreditation Board for Testing and Calibration Laboratories (NABL) provides accreditation to laboratories. Some of these accrediting agencies such as NABH are in turn themselves accredited by ISQua making their standards global in nature.

IPHS are available for subcentres, PHCs, CHCs (ie 30 bedded hospitals), First Referral Units (FRUs), Subdistrict hospitals (51-100 bedded), and district hospitals (separately for those having 101-200 beds, 201-300 beds and 301-500 beds). The standards were introduced in 2007 and revised in 2012. The revisions reflected changing protocols of existing programmes and introduction of new programmes especially for non-communicable diseases (NCDs). These standards have distinction between "minimum assured services" (i.e. essential services) and "desired services". For examples, subcentres have been categorized as type A and B depending upon whether facilities for conducting deliveries are available or not. Accordingly, type B subcentres should essentially have one extra Auxiliary Nurse Midwife (ANM). Apart from human resources, IPHS provides suggestion on layout indicating the space for the building and other infrastructure facilities, list of equipment, furniture and drugs. The document also mentions a Model Citizen's Charter for appropriate information to the beneficiaries, grievance redressal and constitution of Village Health Sanitation and Nutrition Committee, as well as monitoring process and quality assurance mechanism. States and Union Territories (UTs) are expected to adopt these guidelines to improve the quality of care being provided by their respective health facilities and bring them all at par.

NABH was established by QCI in 2002. Its standards are divided into 10 chapters reflecting 10 dimensions of quality. The process of accreditation by NABH includes the following –

- Intention of accreditation by the healthcare organization
- Seeking Application form from QCI
- Self-assessment and scoring by the organization
- Gap-analysis by the organization
- Correction of the gaps
- Application for pre-assessment by NABH
- Pre-assessment survey
- Final assessment by NABH
- Identification of quality gaps
- Correction of gaps
- Gap Analysis by assessors
- Time-frame for gap-completion
- NABH assessment
- NABH accreditation

Kayakalp initiative and Mera Aspatal (My Hospital) initiatives can be considered as benchmarking standards in public health facilities of India. While Kayakalp initiative has ushered in hygiene and cleanliness revolution and is part of the government of India's vision of Swachh Swasth Sarvatra (Everywhere Clean and Healthy), Mera Aspatal initiative dwells mainly on patient satisfaction. Under Kayakalp scheme, similar public health facilities (PHCs to medical colleges) are grouped together and assessed on predefined quality dimensions. The best facilities in each segment are given cash awards. A considerable proportion of the cash award has to be distributed among best-performing healthcare personnel from the winner facilities. The aim of such cash awards and recognitions is to motivate the health management as well as workers to strive for quality improvement. Innovations in patient-engagement and quality care is given extra marks under this scheme. Under Mera Aspatal initiatives, all visitors to the participating health facilities are telephonically requested to provide their opinion on their level of satisfaction with the care they received. Dissatisfied clients are further probed to identify the areas of care lacking in satisfactory services. The reports of these surveys are shared with the health facilities on a monthly basis. The facilities are expected to conduct root-cause analysis of areas having high dissatisfaction ratings.

Chapter 13

Financial Management in Hospitals

Hemant Joshi

CMA, Sr Practice Lead, Infosys BPM Limited

Dr Arti Gupta

Assistant Professor, Community and Family Medicine,

All India Institute of Medical Sciences Mangalagiri, AP

"The first wealth is health." These words, spoken by Ralph Waldo Emerson in 1860, enlarged the meaning of wealth. Empirically, it is proven that healthy people are likely to contribute more than those who are unhealthy, to the building of the economy and nation — as being in good health improves their chances of employability. A robust healthcare system plays significant role in maintaining the health of people. Hospitals are one of the key institutions in health care system which are established to deliver the health care services. Hence, it is imperative that hospitals are economically sound to provide and sustain the various healthcare services for which they are established. Therefore, the primary goals of financial management at hospitals will be to keep hospitals economically viable and same time ensure that health care services offered by them are affordable and meet quality standards. In a developing and populous country like India, financial management further assumes more importance due to paucity of resources and our growing population.

This chapter introduces the health care professionals to the financial aspects of management of hospitals. It provides the understanding of different methods of recording the financial transactions, nature of revenue and costs, introduction to the concept of responsibility centres, various budgetary methods, what performance measures can be used to measure financial effectiveness, variance analysis and finally touches upon role of technology in managing accounting and financial affairs. Attempt has been made to explain the necessary concepts and its application in simple language while avoiding technical jargons.

Recording of Financial Transactions

All financial transactions can be recorded using two methods – cash basis and accruals basis. The main difference between these two methods of recording of financial transactions is in the timing of recognising the expenses and incomes while preparing income and expenditure account and balance sheet. In cash basis of accounting, expenses are recognised only when they are paid in cash or through the bank account of the organisation; similarly, income is recognised only when received in cash or in the bank account of the organisation. The period for which such expense or income is accrued, is not relevant. The accruals basis of accounting, however, does take into consideration the period for which expense or income pertains to, irrespective of whether such expense has been paid out or not and similarly whether such income has been received or not.

Let's take an example to illustrate the two concepts. Let's assume that a hospital's accounting year is from April to March. For the sake of simplicity, assume that the only expenses are the salaries of the staff and the only income is, monthly donations from government or a corporate body. The hospital pays salaries to the tune of Rs 1,00,000.00 per month and it receives Rs 1,50,000.00 as donation per month. Further, let us assume that the hospital pays salaries on the 5th of every month for the previous month and receives donations on the 10th of every month for the month under consideration.

How salary and donations have been recognised

Salary is recognised for only 11 months for the financial year because for March 2020 salary would have been paid on 5th April 2020. Accordingly, salary paid on 5th April 2020 will not be recognised as expense for financial year ending 31st March 2020. It will be recognised in the month of April for financial year ending 31st March 2021. So, total salary recognised is Rs 1,00,000 x 11 = Rs 11,00,000.00

Revenue is received for 12 months because every month, donation is received on the 10th of the month. From April to March, the hospital would have received donation of Rs. 1,50,000 each month (on the 10th day of each month). Accordingly, revenue is Rs 1,50,000 X 12 = Rs 18,00,000.00

Cash basis of accounting

Income & expenditure account for the year ended 31st March 2020		
		Amount - INR
	Receipts - donations	18,00,000.00
Less:	Salary to staff	11,00,000.00
	Excess of income over expenditure	**7,00,000.00**

How salary and donations have been recognised

Salary is recognised for 12 months for the financial year because the relevant point for recognition is the period for which salary pertains to (and not when it is actually paid). Though for March 2020, salary would have been paid on 5th April 2021, but since it pertains to March 2020, it is recognised as an expense for financial year ending 31st March 2020. So, total salary recognised is Rs 1,00,000 x 12 = Rs 12,00,000.00

Revenue i.e., donations should be recognised for all the 12 months as per month donation is receivable. Date of actual receipt does not matter though in this example, it is received. Revenue for the financial year ending 31st March 2020 is Rs 1,50,000 X 12 = Rs 18,00,000.00

Financial Management in Hospitals

Accrual basis of accounting

		Amount - INR
Income and expenditure account for the year ended 31st March 2020		
	Receipts - donations	18,00,000.00
Less:	Salary to staff	12,00,000.00
	Excess of income over expenditure	**6,00,000.00**

From the above illustration, one can observe that excess of income over expenditure for the same financial year is different under both methods of recognising the expenses and revenues.. An obvious question to ponder is, which method of accounting to recognise and record expense and revenue should be adopted? The answer is usually guided by the policy of the organisation and applicable statutory provisions. However, the general rule is that if the organisation has large scale operations, then accruals basis of accounting should be adopted.

Nature of Revenue and Costs

All the financial transactions of on organisation are finally reflected either of the two statements – income and expenditure statement or balance sheet. For organisations which consider earning profits to be their main objective, income and expenditure statement is known by another name — profit and loss account. Income and expenditure account or statement is used in context of not-for-profit organisations.

Income and expenditure account or statement shows transactions which are revenue in nature, while balance sheet shows transactions which are capital in nature. Hence, it is important to know how to differentiate between revenue and capital nature of financial transactions. The table below can be of help to identify whether a financial transaction (whether receipt or expenditure) is of revenue nature or of capital nature.

	Revenue	**Capital**
Receipts	Recurring frequency	Non recurring frequency
	Received for rendering services or providing goods from recipient of such services/goods	Received to finance the fixed assets from owners or long-term loan providers or donors
	Helps to cover the day-to-day operational expenses	Helps to increase the capacity to service or produce more
	Shown in oncome statement under incomes	Shown in balance sheet under capital
Expenditure	Recurring frequency	Non recurring frequency
	Benefit obtained from such expenditure is for short term only	Benefit obtained from such expenditure is available for long term
	Incurred for day-to-day operational activities	Helps for increasing the existing capacity to service or produce more or add new capacity
	Shown in oncome statement under expenditure	Shown in balance sheet under Fixed Assets

Consider the expenditure incurred to pay salary to hospital staff. To determine whether it is revenue expenditure or capital expenditure, we can refer to the table above. This will reveal that staff salary is recurring in nature i.e., it is paid every month, it is paid so that health professional can provide medical services to patients and such medical services are part of the day-to-day operational activities in a hospital. Hence, we can classify salary of hospital staff as revenue expenditure. Accordingly, it will be shown under heading expenditure in income and expenditure account. Consider another example where a hospital has purchased 100 more beds. This expenditure is not incurred very frequently, such newly purchased beds can be used for long term and it has the impact of enhancing the existing capacity of hospital to service more patients. Accordingly, it is a capital expenditure. Similarly, we can determine the revenue or capital nature of receipts from patients for examining them and receipts from a donor to build new hospital building.

	Cost Center	Revenue Center	Profit Center	Investment Center
What managers / supervisors manages	Cost only	Generates revenue	Earns profit. Incurs cost and generates revenue also.	Funds capex
Objective of responsibility center	Minimization of expenses	Maximization of revenues	Maximization of profits	Building capacity

All revenue nature items, whether income or expenditure, is reported in the income and expenditure statement while all capital nature items, whether income or expenditure is reported in the balance sheet. Note that income and expenditure statement reports what kinds of income have been earned and what expenditure has been incurred during the period of reporting (say – month, quarter or half yearly or yearly). It also shows the net result of the same.

Responsibility Centres

A responsibility centre in an operational unit to which specific functions or activities can be assigned to. Such specific functions or activities has common or similar attributes. Each responsibility centre will have its own objectives and set of goals to achieve, though such objective and goals will always be subordinate to the overall mission and objectives of the hospital. Broadly four types of responsibility centers can be visualised – (a) cost centre (b) revenue centre (c) profit centre and (d) investment centre. The following section provides a summary of what these responsibility centres stands for:

Responsibility Centre: Classification and Key Features

From a financial management perspective, the understanding of the concept of responsibility centres is critical as it can help hospitals to set targets for hospital managers and other management leaders like departmental heads, for units or areas which are under their span of influence and hence achievable.

In practice, the same unit can be entrusted with task of earning revenue and will be also incurring costs and hence will be set up as both cost centre and revenue centre. For example, running a pathology lab.

Budgetary Control

The next step in establishing financial management is to prepare budgets for the responsibility centers, which normally represent departments or activities. A budget in its most simple term is a statement of income or expenses or both, which an organisation plans to earn and spend over a specific period. Budgets are an important tool for management to exercise control over expenditure and revenue. Periodic variance analysis i.e., comparison of budgets with actuals enable management to assess what is going right and what not. This can enable them to take timely corrective actions. While preparing budget level of activity and nature of cost must be analysed. Expenses and incomes normally will fluctuate with level of activity and, hence, a budget must consider various levels of activities and understanding the nature of expenses and income into fixed and variable can help to increase the accuracy of budgeted amount (when compared against actuals).

There exist several approaches for budgeting. Below section provides a high level of understanding of such approaches along with pros and cons of same.

Fixed Budget: It refers to a budget which has been prepared for a single level of activity. For example, a hospital may prepare a budget anticipating that in forthcoming financial year it will service or treat 1,00,000 patients. Accordingly, it will budget various expenses and income considering this count of patients. Fixed budgets should be avoided unless there is 100 per cent certainty that there will not be significant deviation in the activity level. If there is significant variation in the activity level, such a budget has no or very limited utility from financial control perspective.

Flexible Budget: Though such budgets are initially prepared for a certain level of activity, they can vary according to the changes in actual level of activity for financial control purposes. For doing so, it is very important that one has clear understanding of what costs are variable and with respect to what and which costs are fixed and up to what activity level or time period they don't change. Once this knowledge and understanding is there, it is easy to prepare a budget for different activity levels and to ascertain what the budgeted numbers would have been for actual level.

Flexible budgets enable one to have a more objective performance evaluation as the budgeted figures for actual activity level, while conducting a variance analysis, are compared against actual figures rather than the initial budgeted figures which may have become irrelevant due to changes in activity level. However, classifying expenses into variable and fixed may be a difficult task to do.

Incremental Budget: As the name itself suggests, such a budget is incremental over the previous period's budgeted or actual figures. The preparer starts with taking the previous period budget or actuals; the same is then adjusted to cover for things which such a budget did not cover but are now known or are now planned out. For instance, preparer may take last period's actual figure and adjust it inflation and compensation costs of hiring more staff.

Incremental budget has the advantage of being easy and quick to prepare, while such a budget also comes with the problem of any existing inefficiency getting passed on from one budgeting period to the next budgeting period.

Rolling Budget: When a budget is kept updated by addition of another period (say month or quarter) when the earliest period has ended, such a budget is termed as rolling budget. Such a budget also offers the opportunity to update or revise the budgeted figures for the remaining period. For example, a hospital has finalised its budgets for Q1, Q2, Q3 and Q4 for the financial year 2020. When Q1 of 2020 ends, it will add one more quarter i.e,. Q1 of 2021 so that at any point of time budget is available for all the four quarters. Also, it may revise the budgeted figure for Q2, Q3 and Q4 of 2020 while it adds Q1 of 20X1.

Rolling budgets will ensure that, at any point of time, budget figures are current and any new information and data are factored into budgets as and when such information is available. This makes them a good tool to exercise financial control where forecasts and estimation about costs and revenue is difficult to make with desired accuracy. However, preparing a rolling budget is an ongoing exercise and takes good amount of time and efforts.

Activity Based Budgeting (ABB) This kind of budgeting leverages the data and information produced by activity-based costing (ABC) to freeze the budget figures. Once budgeted activity levels are freezed by management, activity rates per unit are used to ascertain the budgeted figures for such freezed activity level.

Since ABB uses ABC, it will be helpful to understand how costing is ascertained under ABC method or technique. ABC has three broad or main steps:

Step 1: Create 'cost pools' which represents activities grouped on basis of how they are driven. For example, for a hospital OPD and OT can be cost pools.

Step 2: Identify cost drivers for each cost pool. Cost drivers triggers the costs to be incurred. For example, in OPD time spent by doctors (whether patients are more or less) will cause salary expenses to be incurred.

Step 3: Compute the cost per unit. Assume that an OPD has 10 doctors and their salary cost is Rs 10,00,000 per month and average number of patients per month is 10,000. Cost per patient is Rs 100.00

Now, if the budget for next year is serve 12,000 patients i.e., to see 20 per cent more patients then the current level, the hospital will have to budget Rs 12,00,000.00 (12000 x 12) and will have hire more doctors.

ABB produces more accurate budgeted figures. It also enables the management to know what drives costs in the organisation; however, this kind of budgeting is complex and requires very deep knowledge of business operations.

Zero Base Budgeting (ZBB): It is a method of budgeting which requires each cost element in budget to be justified as if the activity or area to which this cost relates to is being performed for the first time. In ZBB, various activities compete for getting funds allocation from the budget. As such, it is very important for each activity to justify why it should be performed. The most common method to provide the justification for why an activity should be performed is to do the cost benefit analysis (CBA). Activities for which costs outweigh benefits are not considered for allocation of funds from the budget. For all activities for whom value of benefits outweigh costs are ranked as per cost benefit ratio – value of benefits/cost. Activities with higher cost-benefit ratio are ranked higher and are allocated funds from budgets.

For organisations like hospitals run by the government, which does not have the profit motive, quantification of benefits can be a challenge. In such situation, benefits should be quantified as number of patients to be served multiplied by estimated savings to such patients. This approach helps to compute the cost benefit ratio.

Given that most of the patients who come to avail services of hospitals run or aided by government are from economically poor strata, value of such benefits is more than what is being captured by the approach suggested above. If such a value can be captured for ZBB, it can enhance its accuracy — though for all practical purposes, the suggested approach to capture the value of benefits works well.

ZBB helps to allocate the funds where the impact will be maximum and hence helps to increase effectiveness of the organisation. It also promotes efficiency as activities which has low cost-benefit ratio are not taken up for execution. While benefits of implementing ZBB are large, it is complex, time consuming and may focus on short-term goals only.

Variance Analysis

In its simplest form, variance analysis is an investigation between budgeted or planned figure actuals. It is a powerful tool to control and manage the financial affairs of the organisation. When actual costs are less than budgeted costs, it is termed as favourable variance and is indicative of good performance and, when actual costs are more than budgeted cost, it is termed as adverse variance and is a pointer of bad performance. Once the variances for different items of expenditure have been computed, it is important to find out what caused the variances especially the adverse variances. Investigating the reasons will be of help to the organisation to take steps to prevent such variance in future.

Since investigating the variance requires considerable time, it is highly recommended to set the cut-off above which variance will be investigated. This will enable the organisation to focus on material variance only. Such cut-off is often set as a per cent of the actual cost or absolute amount which is lower. Any variance equal to or above it must be investigated for reasons and steps must be taken to prevent such adverse variance from repeating again.

For example, an organisation has set the cut off for investigating the variance as 5 per cent or Rs 10,000 whichever is less. When it performed variances analysis it was ascertained that compensation costs have adverse variance of Rs 5,00,000. Budgeted compensation cost was Rs 25,00,000 while the actual compensation cost was Rs 30,00,000.

To benefit from variance analysis two things are must – accuracy of figures being compared and commitment to take corrective action.

An accurate budget, which reflects the level of activity and accordingly the budgeted expenses and incomes and accurate recording of actual expenses and incomes in the income statement is the first 'must' requirement. Unless the budgeted figure does not reflect the level of activity and income and expenses corresponding to it and income and expenditure statement does not accurately record the actual incomes and expenses comparing them and then using the variance for financial management is of no or very little use.

Equally important is commitment on the part of the management to act upon the adverse variance which are significant or material in nature. Unless there is some concrete action to ensure that such adverse variances are prevented in future, carrying out variance analysis is of no use. Variance analysis must be backed with management action.

Which budgeting technique to use?

Having discussed various approaches towards budgeting, and understanding the pros and cons of each, the question is, how does one select the most appropriate budgeting technique? To answer this question, one must be able to answer following three key secondary questions:

1. Main objective of organisation:

    Is it to earn profits or provide goods and services to the society especially those sections of society who cannot afford it or do breakthrough research?

2. Sources of funding for the operations:

    Whether a significant proportion of expenditure is funded by government or recovered from those who utilise the output i.e., goods and services of the organisation? What is the funding requirement of the organisation – few lakhs or hundreds of crores?

Answers to the above questions can be helpful in selecting the appropriate budgeting technique for the organisation.

An organisation, like a government run or aided hospital, which is primarily funded by the government and has main objective of servicing the needy and has small scale operations, may prefer to adopt the incremental budget. In contrast, if the same hospital grows and has large scale operations, it will benefit more from ABB. Similarly, an institution, which exists to do breakthrough research, will benefit from ZBB.

Performance Indicators

Before we go further, it is important to get an idea of what performance is all about. Performance is the progress made with respect to the achievement of mission, objectives, goals or functions to perform for which the organisation exists. All organisations can be broadly be divided into two categories — ones which exists or functions for earning profit and ones which exist or function to serve without any profit motive. Knowing the reason for why an organisation has been established is key to knowing what performance can mean to it. For example, an organisation which has earning profits as its mission will focus on profits, return on investment and cash flows, etc., while an organisation which exists to service people or for a social cause like eradicating polio will focus on how many people it has served and/or how many people have been benefited by its service and what the value of such benefit is to them.

Performance indicators tell one about the 'health' of the organisation. They can reveal how profitable, efficient, economic and effective an organisation is. Therefore, when assessing the health of the organisation, it is important to know what performance indicators should be used. Referring to wrong performance indicators will provide incorrect assessment and will not be helpful to understand whether the organisation is performing well or not. The following points must be considered while selecting the performance indicators to be used for assessing the performance of the organisation.

1. Performance indicators should measure the progress made towards achievement of the mission or objectives of the organisation.
2. No single performance indicator can summarise the performance of the organisation therefore more than one performance indicators should be used to assess performance.

3. Performance indicators to be used should be mix of financial and non-financial indicators.

4. To deal with unexpected or emergency, new performance indicator should be developed and reported. Once such situation is over use of performance indicator developed specifically to report on such emergency can be discarded.

5. While computing the performance indicators, consistency should be maintained in terms of methodology used. If consistency is not maintained, comparing of performance with previous periods will be of no use.

Mission and Performance Indicators

Mission of Organisation and Performance Indicator to Refer to	Earning Profits	Serving Society
Main Performance Indicators	Financial	Non-financial
Additional Performance Indicator	Non-financial	Financial

While each organisation depending upon its mission will focus on performing well on its main performance indicators, it will, at the same time, have to consider its performance on additional performance indicators. If the organisation fails to do so, it will be difficult for it to maintain its performance on main performance indicators.

For example, let's say, an organisation which seeks to maximise profits for its shareholders is consistently earning increasing profits (main financial indicator, which is financial in nature) while the customer satisfaction ratings (additional performance indicator which is non-financial in nature) are dipping over the years. Dropping of customers satisfaction rating year after year, will erode customer base and will ultimately wipe out profits. Hence, to maintain the increase in profits, this organization must focus on improving the customer satisfaction rating.

Let's take another example and this time we will consider an organisation whose mission is to service people in rural area in healthcare field (say an hospital). This hospital has been providing healthcare services to an increasing number of rural people (main financial indicator, which is non-financial in nature) but its expense over income, also referred to as deficit (additional performance indicator, which is financial in nature) is also increasing with each year. Just looking at the number of people served each year, one may conclude that it is performing well, but when this is read with the deficit it has over the years, its becomes obvious that the hospital may get closed down in the near future.

The previous two examples highlight that irrespective of whether an organization exists for earning profits or for servicing people, it must measure and report a mix of financial and non-financial performance measures for an accurate assessment of its performance. The following table provides some examples of performance indicators – main and additional, which organisation can set and measure for achieving its mission and objective. In this example, the organisation whose mission is to serve society is assumed to be a hospital largely funded by the government.

Examples of Performance Indicators

Mission of Organisation and Performance Indicators	Earning Profit	Serving Society
Main Performance Measures	Operating cash flows Profits — gross and net Return on Investment (RoI) Profit Before Interest Tax (PBIT) Profit After Tax (PAT) Economic Value Added (EVA)	Patients attended/Day Patients attended/Doctor Percentage of Patients Treated Successfully
Additional Performance Measures	Percentage of Market Share Change in Percentage of Market Share Customer Satisfaction Rating Employee Satisfaction Rating	Excess of Income over Expenditure/Deficit Percentage of Increase In Donations/Funds Percentage of Reduction in Costs

Note: Performance indicators in blue and green are financial and non-financial in nature, respectively.

Technological Advances in Managing Financial Affairs

Technology has practically touched all spheres of accounting and financial management making it more simple, more accurate and comprehensive while increasing predictability and creating financial models which can be used to manage costs and income more efficiently and effectively. This section introduces the reader to how advancements in technology are shaping the accounting and financial management at organisations.

Accounting which primarily concerns itself with the recording of financial transactions has traditionally been a manual and time-consuming exercise. Another challenge with such forms of accounting was that, it has little insight to offer about the performance of the organisation. A lot of data was required to be processed outside the accounting package so that reports could be prepared for the management to review performances. Accounting data being historical in nature has very limited usage in financial management, especially in budgeting and forecasting. Another inherent limitation of accounting is that it fails to capture the non-financial which, for organisations with no profit motive, is key to measuring and assessing performance.

The latest accounting and Enterprise Resource Planning (ERP) packages have integrated accounting with financial management to a great extent. Nowadays, ERPs like SAP, Oracle and others provides lot of flexibility to automate a large part of recording of financial transactions. This has reduced the cost of running the accounting department within organisations. Such ERP packages also provide many reporting features which can be of great help in managing financial affairs of the organisation. For example, cash flow statement can be extracted for any period – day, week, month, quarter or year. Not only this, at the mere click of a mouse, management can run reports to see what the major expense heads are, what the variance between actual and budgeted expenses heads is, what the net result of the income earned and expenditure incurred for the period is (again, period can be day, week, month, quarter or year) and balance sheet at any point of time. It can also provide trend analysis of income and expenditure. Another key feature of such ERPs is that they offer the ease of preparing budgets and doing forecasting, along with variance analysis at the level of the responsibility centre, thereby, making financial management more accurate and faster.

While advantages of managing the financial affairs using an ERP might seem to be panacea for all the finance administration-related issues, the same is not the case. First, deploying an ERP can cost large amount of money which an organisation may not afford. Second, ERP implementation can take months and subsequent to that, there may be issues in terms of how correct the data produced by ERP is, owing to technical and other issues (note that it may not be an issue with the ERP but with the way in which it is configured). Third, working with ERP requires training and specialised knowledge. Hiring of people with such skills may cost more. Fourth, there may be other maintenance and upgradation cost associated with ERP. Apart from these four major hurdles, another key issue which may come up pertains to technical issues which may surface from time to time.

Having an overview of benefits and costs associated with ERP may put the management of an organisation in a dilemma about whether to implement an ERP or not. The answer to this question is not straightforward and will depend on many factors. The first important factor is the scale of financial transactions of the organisation. Managing large number of transactions manually or even with some basic accounting package may not be the most economical way. The second key factor is the cost of the ERP – one needs to determine whether one-time funding and funding for running it can be secured or not. These two factors are the main determinants of whether an organisation can and should implement ERP. Another consideration, apart from managing financial affairs, is whether ERP facilitates other tasks like managing patients records and other details, whether it can do resource planning in term shift and patient allocation etc.

Summary

Managing financial affairs of an organisation starts with recording and understanding the nature of financial transactions. Performance, especially the financial aspect, must be reviewed considering the mission or objective of the organisation. Whether an organisation has been established for earning profit or for serving society, will greatly determine what performance measures should be tracked and managed by the leadership of the organisation. It is important for an organisation to select the appropriate mix of financial and non-financial performance measures to track and report. Various financial management techniques like budgeting, forecasting, variance analysis and creation of responsibility centres among others can play an important role in making an efficient and effective use of the organisation's resources. Selection of appropriate form technique for financial management will be influenced by many considerations and careful evaluation of them is recommended. Advent of EPP has made financial administration easier and more efficient, though there is a cost attached to it. Organisation should do comparative analysis of benefits and associated costs pertaining to ERP implementation along with considerations of other relevant factors like, whether ERP can support other functions to decide on this subject.

CHAPTER 14

Leadership in Health Management

Dr. Sidharth Sekhar Mishra,

Assistant Professor

International Institute of Health Management Research, New Delhi

INTRODUCTION

This unit covers the leadership and team building. We start with definition of leadership and importance of team building. This is followed by classification of leadership which consists of executive appointed leadership, leadership appointed by the group, self-appointed leader etc. Then we also deal with democratic, authoritarian and institutional leaderships. Then we take up the various factors constituting leadership and within this we discuss the leader, followers, communication and situations. Then we take up characteristics of leadership within which we discuss the interpersonal skills, communication skills, values, organizational consciousness etc. Then we take up the tasks of leadership within which we deal with confidence, flexibility, creative skills, achieving results etc. This is followed by approach of leadership and this is discussed in terms of the trait approach, authoritarian approach, Likert system approach, managerial grid approach etc.

Objectives

After completing this unit, you will be able to:

- Define leadership;
- Understand the types of leadership;
- Describe the approaches to leadership;
- Explain the tasks of leadership; and

Definition of Leadership

There are many definitions of leadership:

I. "A simple *definition of leadership* is that leadership is the art of motivating a group of people to act towards achieving a common goal."

This definition of leadership captures the leadership essentials of inspiration and preparation. Effective leadership is based upon ideas, but will not happen unless those ideas can be communicated to others in a way that engages them.

II. Put even more simply, the leader is the "inspiration and director of the action". He is the person in the group that possesses the combination of personality and leadership skills that makes others want to follow his direction.

III. Peter Drucker defined leader as someone who has followers. To gain followers requires influence but does not exclude the lack of integrity in achieving this. Indeed, it can be argued that several of the world's greatest leaders have lacked integrity and have adopted values that would not be shared by many people today.

IV. In the 21 Irrefutable Laws of Leadership, John Maxwell sums up his definition of leadership as "leadership is influence - nothing more, nothing less." This moves beyond the position defining the leader, to looking at the ability of the leader to influence others, that is, both those who would consider themselves followers, and those outside that circle. Indirectly, it also builds in leadership character, since without maintaining integrity and trustworthiness, the capability to influence will disappear.

V. Warren Bennis' definition of leadership is focused much more on the individual capability of the leader. He defined leadership as a function of knowing oneself, having a vision that is well communicated, building trust among colleagues, and taking effective action to realize one's own leadership potential.

VI. According to Pigors, "Leadership is a process of control in which by the assumption of superiority a person or group regulates the activities of others for purposes of his own choosing."

Classification of Leadership

Classification of Leadership Based on		
Origin	**Purpose**	**Nature**
Executive Appointed	Intellectual	Authoritarian
Leader Appointed	Artistic	Democratic
Self-Appointed	Executive	Institutional
		Dominant
		Expert
		Persuasive

A. Basis of Origin

I. Executive Appointed Leadership

The person is appointed by the executive and the leadership stems from the office or post to which the person is appointed by the executive. The class of government officers is of this type.

II. Leader Appointed by the Group

These leaders are elected by the group. Public leaders of panchayats, local groups, the Lok Sabha and Rajya Sabha are elected by the group.

III. Self-Appointed Leader

There are some leaders whose authority derives neither from the executive nor the group because it is not vested in them by these groups. They advance because of their individual qualities and having attained the central position, lead the people. They are recognized as such because of their qualities.

B. Basis of Purpose

I. Intellectual Leadership

This leadership is in the intellectual field. In the field of philosophy, science etc. the greatest thinkers can be said as intellectual leaders because they show the way and the others follow them.

II. Artistic Leadership

This leadership is in the field of art, only the great artists can provide the leadership.

III. Executive Leadership

This type of leadership is in the sphere of administration, it is the authoritative personality who becomes the leader.

C. Basis of Nature

I. Authoritarian Leadership

The authoritarian leader is an individual who likes to assert his authority. He does not consult any one in taking decisions and leads by creating fear into the hearts of his followers and subordinates. He keeps all his authority in his hands and appoints reliable subordinates at crucial position. Leader of this kind is an officer and an authoritarian. He prefers to issue orders and punishes who disobey him.

II. Democratic Leadership

This type of leader is of a democratic mould in his thoughts, modes of action and conduct. He takes advice from every one and is always anxious to enlist the cooperation of any one who is willing to give it. His leadership is based upon sympathy, belief and affection. He does not call himself a leader and neither does he take all the authority into his own hands.

III. Institutional Leadership

There are some individuals who occupy the highest post. His orders are appreciated and implemented because of the authority vested in his chair. The institutional leader is not leader but the officiating head.

IV. Dominant Leader

The leader is so called because he maintains a relation of authority and dominance with his followers or subordinates. He does not rule over them. However successful he may appear because of his power and authority.

V. Expert Leadership

A Leader of this type does not put any premium on maintaining social contact with their followers, understanding them or even knowing their thoughts. People come to them for advice from time to time, respect their opinions.

Expert leaders are experts, and should not be considered as leaders. The basis of their contact with their followers and subordinates is their special ability and efficiency.

VI. **Persuasive Leadership**

The persuasive leaders win the heart of their followers and do their best to maintain the closest social contact with them. These are the real leaders. It is only this kind of individual who really exhibits all the qualities of leadership.

The overall picture reveals a variety of leadership style and their characteristics which we have to know about leadership. In context of organizational setting only three major leadership style we can discuss here. These are autocratic, democratic and lassiez- faire leadership style and each of which have some significant features.

Salient features of Types of Leadership

Autocratic/Authoritarian/ Production Centered leadership	Democratic/Employee centered leadership	Laissez-Faire leadership
<ul><li>Exercises close supervision.</li><li>Makes most decision himself.</li><li>Emphasizes on production.</li><li>Permits little or no initiative to subordinates.</li><li>Gives detailed instructions and directions.</li><li>Subordinates' suggestions and ideas are not allowed.</li><li>Authority oriented.</li></ul>	<ul><li>Delegate authority and responsibility.</li><li>Manages through objectives.</li><li>Permits initiative and responsibility.</li><li>Seeks and encourages employees' suggestions.</li><li>Participative decision-making.</li><li>Emphasizes production as well as employee satisfaction</li></ul>	<ul><li>Emphasizes neither production, nor employee satisfaction.</li><li>It is directionless.</li><li>Employees are left to drifting.</li></ul>
Transformational leadership Besides this, there is another type of leadership, named transformational leadership. It is defined as leadership that goes beyond normal expectations by inspiring new ways of thinking, stimulating learning experiences and transmitting a sense of mission. These leaders are sometimes called super leaders. They act in such a way that it is possible to transform average organization into exceptional organization.		

Factors Affecting Leadership Traits

I. Leader

The leader must have an honest understanding of who he is, what he knows, and what he can do. Also, note that it is the followers, not the leader or someone else who determines if the leader is successful. If they do not trust or lack confidence in their leader, then they will be uninspired. To be successful the leader must convince his followers, that he is worthy of being followed.

II. Followers

Different people require different styles of leadership. For example, a new hire requires more supervision than an experienced employee. A person who lacks motivation requires a different approach than one with a high degree of motivation. The leader must therefore know his people. The fundamental starting point is having a good understanding of human nature, such as needs, emotions, and motivation. The leader must know his employees and their attributes.

III. Communication

The leader leads through two-way communication. He has to set the example and communicate to them that he would not ask them to perform anything that he would not be willing to do. What and how the leader communicates either builds or harms the relationship between the leader and his employees.

IV. Situation

"All situations are different" - What one does in one situation will not always work in another. The leader must use his judgment to decide the best course of action and the leadership style needed for each situation.

Also note that the *situation* normally has a greater effect on a leader's action than his or her traits. This is because while traits may have an impressive stability over a period of time, they have little consistency across situations. This is why a number of leadership scholars think the *Process Theory of Leadership* is a more accurate than the *Trait Theory of Leadership*.

Various forces will affect these four factors. Examples of forces are the leader's relationship with his seniors, the skill of his followers, the informal leaders within his organization, and how his organization is organized.

Characteristics of Leadership

In business, leadership is welded to performance. Those who are viewed as effective leaders are those who increase their company's bottom lines.

Leadership is a process by which a person influences others to accomplish an objective and directs the organization in a way that makes it more cohesive and coherent. Leaders carry out this process by applying their leadership knowledge and skills. This is called *Process Leadership*. However, we know that we have traits that can influence our actions. This is called *Trait Leadership* in that it was once common to believe that leaders were born rather than made.

Leadership is the art of influencing others to direct their will, abilities and efforts to the achievement of leader's goals. In the context of organizations, leadership lies in influencing individual and group effort toward the optimum achievement of organizational objectives.

Leadership focuses on "people" aspect of management and is based on the assumption that organizational effectiveness significantly depends on their motivation, effort and abilities. The human relations movement, beginning with the Hawthorne studies in early thirties, focused on the important role of employee motivation and group norms of organizational success. This led to the recognition of leadership effectiveness as an important determinant of organizational effectiveness.

It is the manager in his leadership role who has to stimulate and inspire the employees to contribute willingly and cooperatively to the optimum achievement of organizational goals. In this context, one important term we can use, i.e., team. Generally, team members support one another. They offer suggestions and give feedback to other members. They may disagree but work to resolve differences and reach consensus. Each and every member of the team trust and support other members.

Anyone who acts as a model to others is often called a "leader". Leadership is attribute of that person who is an ideal for the other members of the group. Leadership is the behavior that affects the behavior of other people, more than their behavior affects that of the leader. In fact, we can say that in every group every member bears some relation to the others and all of them influence and affect each other. Leader leads, suggests, orders and also guides. Other people follow him. We can say that leadership and domination are not the same meaning.

According to MacIver and Page Leadership is the capacity to persuade or to direct man that comes from personal qualities apart from office. It indicates the difference between leadership and office. An individual does not become a leader only by occupying an office which carries responsibility. It is a matter of secondary importance that his important office is of assistance to him in his endeavor to become a leader. Leadership depends upon the individual qualities of the person and not the office that he holds. Leadership is the term which denotes the behavior or functions of the leader. The leader affects the individual in such a way they surrender themselves and follow his dictates.

Characteristics of leadership are as follows:

1. Leader is the total ideal of the followers.
2. Leader is shown regard.
3. Leader and the followers influence each other.
4. Leader's order is a command.
5. Leader controls the other member of the group.
6. Leader determines the group's conduct.
7. Leader is a respected and revered person.

Listed below are eight leadership characteristics:

I. Interpersonal Skills

Leaders that have earned the trust and respect of their followers can use this trust to move the organization towards the achievements of its goal. These leaders are able to use their interpersonal skills to work through difficult situations and keep peace in their organizations. These individuals are good at listening as well as providing constructive feedback.

II. Communication Skills

Leaders demonstrating communication skills are both good speakers and listeners. Through their words they can help keep the workforce motivated and committed. They also listen to their followers, and ask questions when they want to have a good understanding of what is being expressed.

III. Values

Leaders must also value the diversity of a workforce, and understand that a diverse group of employees will bring a broader perspective to the organization. They will treat followers with the respect they deserve, and do not display favoritism. They operate with a high level of ethics, which becomes an example for others to follow.

IV. **Organizational Consciousness**

Leadership characteristics sometimes go beyond personal traits, and touch on areas such as organizational consciousness or knowledge. These are leaders that understand what the organization wants to achieve, and know how it can be accomplished. They create networks within the organization to help their groups get work done, and are just as adept at breaking down organizational barriers to progress.

V. **Confidence**

Leaders need to carry themselves with confidence, and should not be afraid to take ownership for both popular and unpopular decisions. They must be able to learn from criticisms, and be often acutely aware of their own shortcomings. Confident leaders are able to maintain a calm demeanor even during emergencies, and this can be contagious when it needs to be.

VI. **Flexibility**

Another important characteristic of leaders is their ability to remain flexible, and adapt their leadership style to meet the demands of the current work environment. They must be able to work with others to meet organizational goals, and shift focus as necessary.

VII. **Creativity Skills**

Leaders demonstrating creativity skills are able to develop innovative solutions to old problems. The diversity they build in their organizations helps them to develop more comprehensive answers to routine questions. Creative leaders are able to translate technical information into solutions that are understood by everyone.

VIII. **Achieving Results**

Leaders just do not set the example for others to follow. They also play a big role in achieving the goals of the organization. Through their leadership skills, they maintain a high level of performance in their organizations, and they are able to help keep their workforce motivated even when faced with a seemingly impossible situation.

Since they have a deep understanding of what an organization needs to accomplish, they are able to quickly identify and solve the important objectives of an organization.

Leadership is much more complex than merely earning a high-status position in a company, and the ability to order people to do things. It is a participative journey that the leader must be willing to walk with others. It is a skill that's acquired over a lifetime, and these characteristics are something we can practice about every day of our life. A great leader is one who learns from his mistakes.

Tasks of Leadership

The principal tasks of leadership are presented below:

1. To recognize that people differ in their motivational pattern.
2. To gain an understanding of group dynamics.
3. To create an environment that produces convergence of individual goals and organizational goals.

4. To stimulate and inspire employees as individuals and group members to make their optimum contribution to organizational efficiency and effectiveness.

5. To make sense of changing environment, interpret it to employees and redirect their efforts to adapt to changing situation.

Approaches of Leadership

The main approaches of leadership are:

1. The trait approach.
2. Approaches based on the use of authority.
3. Likert's approach.
4. The managerial grid approach.
5. The path-goal approach.
6. The contingency approach.
7. The continuum approach.

1. **The Trait Approach**

   The trait approach aims at identifying some unique qualities that would distinguish more effective managers from less effective managers.

2. **The Use of Authority Approach**

   One approach classified managers as democratic, authoritarian and lassiez-faire. The Ohio State University studies identified leadership on two orthogonal dimensions, viz., consideration and initiation. The University of Michigan studies distinguished between production oriented and employee oriented leaders on a simple dimension.

3. **Likert System Approach**

   There are mainly four types of approach. System I is Exploitative Authoritarian system, System II is Benevolent Authoritative system, System III is Consultative and System IV is Participative group leadership. The system IV is most effective for employee need satisfaction as well as optimum organizational performance.

4. **Managerial Grid Approach**

   Leadership style in on a grid with 9-point on the horizontal axis and 9-point on vertical axis. Horizontal axis indicates "Concern for production" and vertical axis indicates "concern for people".

   We can say 1, 1 leadership style is impoverished management with minimum concern for production and minimum concern for people; 9,1 style leader indicates maximum concern for production and minimum concern for people. We can further say that 1,9 style indicates minimum concern for production and maximum concern for people. 9,9 style is most effective because it indicates maximum concern for production and maximum concern for people. In this context it can be said that 5,5 style is recognized as mid-of-the-road style.

5. **Path-Goal Approach**

   Leader's effectiveness depends on his ability to provide opportunities for employee need satisfaction and make need satisfaction contingent on performance effectiveness.

6. **Contingency Approach**

   There are mainly two kinds of behaviour – (i) task-oriented and (ii) people and interpersonal-oriented. What kind of leader will succeed depends on the three situations mainly:

   - Leader's personal relationship with group members.
   - Formal authority of the leader and
   - Degree of task structure.

     Task oriented leaders will be effective when situation is very favorable or very unfavorable. In intermediate situations, people and inter-personal oriented leader will be effective.

7. **Continuum Approach**

   There are mainly seven types of leader's behavior on a continuum. At one end of the continuum, the leader has almost full freedom to make decision and at the other end subordinate group has it. In the middle, both have equal freedom when leader presents tentative decisions subject to change after non-manager input. Mainly the choice of leadership style depends on the situation. On the other hand, manager consider three following factors, viz.,

   - forces within himself,
   - forces in the subordinate and
   - forces in the situation.

"An organization may choose any approach considering the above-mentioned leadership approaches."

References

1. Klingborg DJ, Moore DA, Varea-Hammond S. What is leadership? J Vet Med Educ. 2006 Summer;33(2):280-3. doi: 10.3138/jvme.33.2.280. PMID: 16849311.

2. O'Keeffe DF. Leadership. Curr Opin Obstet Gynecol. 2012 Dec;24(6):436-9. doi: 10.1097/GCO.0b013e328359b605. PMID: 23090618.

3. Low S, Butler-Henderson K, Nash R, Abrams K. Leadership development in health information management (HIM): literature review. Leadersh Health Serv (Bradf Engl). 2019 Sep 26;32(4):569-583. doi: 10.1108/LHS-11-2018-0057. Epub 2019 Sep 20. PMID: 31612782.

4. Harris J, Mayo P. Taking a case study approach to assessing alternative leadership models in health care. Br J Nurs. 2018 Jun 14;27(11):608-613. doi: 10.12968/bjon.2018.27.11.608. PMID: 29894257.

5. Koka S, Baba K, Ercoli C, Fitzpatrick B, Jiang X. Leadership in an academic discipline. J Dent. 2019 Aug;87:40-44. doi: 10.1016/j.jdent.2019.05.020. Epub 2019 May 16. PMID: 31103704.

6. Mansel B. Emotional intelligence is essential to leadership. Nurs Stand. 2017 Jan 18;31(21):29. doi: 10.7748/ns.31.21.29.s28. PMID: 28098012.

7. Roussel L. Leadership's Impact on Quality, Outcomes, and Costs. Crit Care Nurs Clin North Am. 2019 Jun;31(2):153-163. doi: 10.1016/j.cnc.2019.02.003. Epub 2019 Apr 8. PMID: 31047090.

8. Giltinane CL. Leadership styles and theories. Nurs Stand. 2013 Jun 12-18;27(41):35-9. doi: 10.7748/ns2013.06.27.41.35.e7565. PMID: 23905259.

Chapter 15

Biomedical Waste Management

Dr Nabanita Banerjee

Assistant Professor

Maharaja Jitendra Narayan Medical College and Hospital, West Bengal

The Bio Medical Waste Management Rules 2016 define "bio-medical waste" as any waste, which is generated during the diagnosis, treatment or immunisation of human beings or animals or research activities pertaining thereto or in the production or testing of biological or in health camps, including the categories mentioned in Schedule I appended to these rules.

Of the total amount of waste generated by healthcare activities, about 15 per cent is considered hazardous material. In a large tertiary care hospital in India, the waste generated is about **1-2 kg/bed/day.**

Sources of Biomedical Waste

Hospitals, nursing homes, clinics, medical laboratories, medical research centres, blood banks, mortuaries animal houses, waste generated at home when health care is provided to a patient at home (e.g., injection vials, dressing material, etc.).

Types of Biomedical Waste[1]

Infectious waste
Pathological waste
Sharps waste
Chemical waste
Pharmaceutical waste
Cytotoxic waste
Radioactive waste

Effects of Biomedical Waste

1. Exposure to potentially harmful microorganisms
2. Sharps-inflicted injuries: Hepatitis B infections and Hepatitis C infections
3. Toxic exposure to pharmaceutical products (antibiotics and cytotoxic drugs) and mercury or dioxins
4. Chemical burns and thermal injuries
5. Air pollution arising as a result of the release of particulate matter during medical waste incineration (inadequate incineration or the incineration of unsuitable materials)
6. Radiation burns
7. Disposal of untreated health care wastes in landfills can lead to contamination of drinking, surface, and ground waters.

India implemented Biomedical Waste Management Rules in 1998 under Environment Protection Act (EPA), 1986. This was modified several times, such as in 2000, 2003 and 2011. A major change was brought about in the year 2016 with the introduction of new Biomedical Waste Management Rules. Further amended in 2018[1]. This consists of **18 Rules, 4 Schedules and 5 Forms.**

The salient features of the Biomedical Waste Rule 2016 are:

1. The scope of the rules was expanded to include various health camps such as vaccination camps, blood donation camps, and surgical camps.
2. Duties of the occupier of a HCFs have been revised.
3. Biomedical waste has been classified into four categories based on colour-code-type of waste and treatment options.
4. No HCF shall establish on-site BMW treatment and disposal facility if the provision of CBMWTF is present at a distance of 75 kilometres.
5. Standards for emission from incinerators have been modified to be more environmental friendly.

There are four categories of biomedical waste under the new rule, based on the segregation pathway and colour code.

1. Yellow Category
2. Red Category
3. White Category
4. Blue Category.

These categories are further divided as per the type of waste under each category as follows:

Categorisation and Classification of Wastes in Healthcare Facilities

Category	Classification
Yellow	(1) **Human Anatomical Waste**
	(2) **Animal Anatomical Waste**
	(3) **Soiled Waste**
	(4) **Discarded or Expired Medicine**
	(5) **Chemical Waste**
	(6) **Chemical Liquid Waste**
	(7) **Discarded linen, mattresses, beddings contaminated with blood or body fluid, routine mask and gown.**
	(8) **Microbiology, Biotechnology and other clinical laboratory waste (Pre-treated**
Red	Contaminated waste (recyclable)
White	Waste sharps including metals, needles, syringes with fixed needles
Blue	Broken or discarded and contaminated glass including medicine vials and ampoules except those contaminated with cytotoxic wastes.

Steps Involved in Bio-medical Waste Management

1. Segregation,
2. Collection,
3. Pre-treatment,
4. Intramural Transportation and
5. Storage

} Exclusive responsibility of HCF(health care facility)

6. Treatment and Disposal — primarily responsibility of CBWTF operator except for lab and highly infectious waste, which is required to be pre-treated by the HCF.

Segregation

Segregated wastes of different categories need to be collected in identifiable containers.

Category	Colour and Type of Container for Collection
Yellow	Yellow coloured non-chlorinated plastic bags Chemical waste (yellow-e) should be stored in yellow container
Red	Red coloured non chlorinated plastic bags (having thickness equal to more than 50 μ) and containers
White	White coloured translucent, puncture proof, leak proof, temper proof containers
Blue	Puncture proof, leak proof boxes or containers with blue coloured marking

Collection and Storage

- Bio-medical waste should be collected on a daily basis from each ward of the hospital at a fixed time at a fixed interval of time.
- HCF should also ensure disposal of human anatomical waste, animal anatomical waste, soiled waste and biotechnology waste within 48 hours.
- General waste should not be collected at the same time or in the same trolley in which bio-medical waste is collected.

Treatment Options for Bio-medical Waste

Category	Treatment
Yellow	No treatment of waste is required to be carried out at the healthcare facility except pre-treatment (sterilisation) of Yellow (h) category waste by autoclaving/microwaving or sterilise as per WHO Blue book 2014.
Red	Contaminated recyclable waste containing mainly plastics and rubber put in red coloured non chlorinated plastic bags and containers.
White	Collection in puncture proof, leak proof, tamper proof container $\longrightarrow$ handover waste to CBWTF.
Blue (a) Glassware	Dispose of the empty glass bottles by handing over to CBWTF. The residual chemicals in glass bottle should be collected as chemical waste in yellow coloured container/bags and over to CBWTF as yellow (e) waste.
Blue (b)	Dispose of the waste by handing over to CBWTF. In case of no access to CBWTF, metallic body implants should be disinfected and later washed with detergent prior to sending/selling to metal recyclers.

Biomedical Waste Management During Covid-19 Pandemic

1. COVID-19 Isolation Wards:

- Separate colour coded bins/bags/containers in wards and proper segregation of waste as per BMWM Rules, 2016
- Double layered bags (using two bags) for collection of waste from COVID-19 isolation wards
- Collection and storage of biomedical waste separately prior to handing over the same CBWTF
- Dedicated collection bin labelled as "COVID-19" to store COVID-19 waste and kept separately in temporary storage room prior to handing over to CBWTF
- Bags/containers for collecting biomedical waste from COVID-19 wards, should be labelled as "COVID-19 Waste"
- Separate record of waste generated from COVID-19 isolation wards
- Dedicated trolleys and collection bins in COVID-19 isolation wards
- Inner and outer surfaces of containers/trolleys for storage of COVID-19 waste should be disinfected with 1 per cent sodium hypochlorite solution daily
- Dedicated sanitation workers separately for biomedical waste and general solid waste

2. Quarantine Home/Home-care in Covid-19:

- Hand over the yellow bags containing biomedical waste generated there to authorised waste collectors at door steps engaged by local bodies; or
- Deposit biomedical waste in yellow bags at designated deposition centres established by ULBs, or
- Hand over the biomedical waste to waste collector engaged by CBWTF operator at the doorstep

References

1. 'Government of India Ministry of Environment, Forest and Climate Change notification'. *Gazette of India*, *Extraordinary*, Part II, Section 3, Sub-section (i). New Delhi, 28 March 2016.

2. 'Directorate General of Health Services (Ministry of Health & Family Welfare) and Central Pollution Control Board (Ministry of Environment, Forest & Climate Change): Guidelines for Management of Healthcare Waste as per Biomedical Waste Management Rules, 2016'.

3. WHO fact Sheet No 253. 'Waste from Health Care Activities'. Available at http: //www.who.int/media centre/factsheets/fs253/en/. Accessed on 16 February 2021.

4. World Health Organisation. 'Safe Management of Wastes from Healthcare Activities: A Summary'. 2017.

CHAPTER 16

Human Resource Management

Dr. Satabdi Mitra

Assistant Professor, Department of Community Medicine

KPC medical college and hospital, Kolkata, West Bengal

OVERVIEW OF HUMAN RESOURCE MANAGEMENT (HRM), ITS IMPORTANCE AND FUNCTIONING

Human resource management (HRM), a long overlooked matter, is an important prop which acts as a rig of organization. This is the department which deals with most valuable resource starting from its development to maintenance, promotion, increment, transfer, welfare, retention, grievance redressal even initiation and if required, resolution of regulatory actions as well as handling workers' union bodies and court cases.

Human resource management acts as breath of life of the organization and HR department is essentially and intricately related to all its weal and woe. The process of functioning is 'line function' embedded in broad 'staff function'.

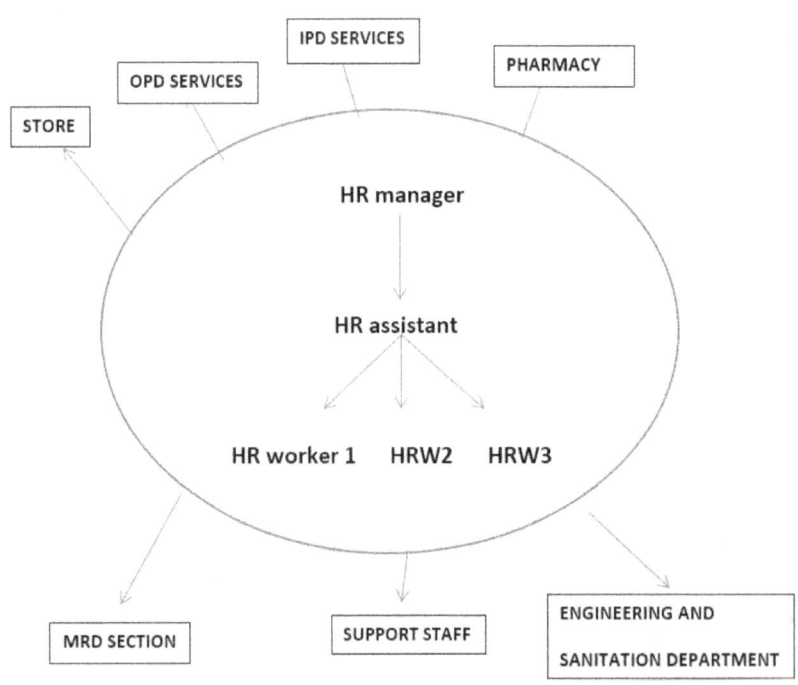

Fig.: Within the circle, the HR in line function, which indicates direct supervision, monitoring and command from higher to lower level staff. Whereas, outside the circle, with all the departments they have supportive role, maintenance of liaison and have advisory role as staff function.

Functions of human resource management

The end-objective of human resource management being to improve the workers, managers and organization, in broad and functions are as follows:

1. Manpower planning
2. Manpower development
   (a) Recruitment
   (b) Training
   (c) Periodic audit
   (d) Job analysis and job enrichment

3. Manpower resourcing
   (a) Lateral entry
   (b) Head hunting
   (c) Retention of employee
   (d) Re-recruitment of retired staff

4. Evaluation of performance
5. Grievance redressal

Recruitment:

The system of recruitment needs determining some basic and essential principles which cannot be violated unless there some extraordinary situation arises. Recruitment aims at ensuring right person to be placed in right position and provided with right compensation.

The process of recruitment is as follow:

1. Analysis of requirement: it consists of detailed chalking out of manpower requirement of the organization and planning according to priority for sequential placement of manpower at various positions.
2. Preparation for recruitment: this is essentially the process of matching 'job description' to 'job specification'. It needs a detailed planning so that potential applicants have a clear idea on expectations from them and that will save time for both applicants and selectors.
3. Inviting applications: the application format should have enough clarity on essential and desirable requirements following existing norms and to be approachable through print and online routes within reasonable time limit.
4. Screening of the applications: a committee with adequate representation of eligible selectors has to prepare a list of candidates to be called for interview. If number of applicants is too much, many a times in first step, ineligible candidates are excluded before reaching to expert selectors.

5. Interview: it is one of the most crucial corner stone in the process of employment as it is the last hatchway the candidate has to pass through. With passage of time, interview process undergoes modifications and it is the competency-based interview that is followed in number of organization. Here the interviewee is given problem-based questions frequently faced in workplace and the selectors assess the ways and aptitude the candidate is opting for.

6. Placement: it is the last part of the recruitment process and it is often the key to improvement of organization of getting satisfied and motivated employees with least employee turnover, absenteeism, employee walkaway etc.

Training:

Once the employees become the part of organization, it is the responsibility of both the employee and employer to work together for progress of the individual and as a whole of the organization. To fulfil it training need to be assessed and accordingly staff training to be conducted.

1. Induction training: for each category of personnel, it is necessary to give induction training for clarifying their roles and responsibilities for the current job and ways to follow for future further improvement. It encourages mingling among staff themselves and being familiar with the organization too.

2. In service training: in order to keep the staff updated on recent advances on the sector and section of his/her work, on-the-job training is very much important. It is especially of tremendous value for ever growing and changing sector like health.

3. Promotional training: some governing bodies keep some of the training needed for further upgradation of position. It is the duty in part of both employee and employer to complete these trainings before attaining eligibility for next level post.

4. Specialized training: for improvement of knowledge and skill, the organization should motivate the employee for taking part in different trainings, courses, conferences, workshops, both on-site and online.

Job enrichment:

It is an emerging concept in human resource management. It aims at 'vertical enlargement' of responsibilities so that talented employees can find out challenges, innovations, satisfaction, and shared decision making opportunities and thereby the organization will grow in breadth and future managerial heads will be identified.

Evaluation of performance:

It is generally called as performance appraisal and its recorded version is named as 'annual confidential reports (ACR)'. The employee in each financial year fill up one form of self-appraisal and in sealed envelope it is sent to the official of higher rank; with comments and marks from reviewing authority it is kept in confidential custody and opened at time of beneficial promotion time.

This age old practice has long been criticized for keeping the employee in dark without any provision of feedback and based on it sixth pay commission recommended for ACR-based increments which because of various reasons was not universally accepted. There are scopes for reformation and refinement of ACR to bring about transparency in it and keeping it above opprobrium of sycophancy.

In order to overcome this, few modifications has been introduced in performance appraisal like as, anniversary system, where employees are appraised on anniversary of employment. There is another system called calendar system. Here all are assessed on single time. One innovative system is 360 degree appraisal. In current medical graduate curriculum it has also been introduced by taking review from employer, immediate supervisor, colleagues and students/clients. This multi-source feedback is especially helpful to assess professional qualities of work.

Challenges of human resource management for an organization

One interesting thing in the world of human resource management is its intrinsic challenges.

1. First and foremost challenge for any organization is to get and maintain a stable and motivated HR team which may act a driving force for it.

2. Staff turnover is another important factor. Once a worker gets accustomed to a workplace, on getting transferred becomes a difficulty for both sides.

3. Workplace harassment up to level of bullying or gender-based harassment, if not addressed by zero tolerance by employer, turns to evil for the organization body too.

4. Unclear system of promotion, increment etc. also creates employee dissatisfaction and ultimately affects adversely.

5. Non-working or sleeping grievance redressal system also becomes a major challenge for organization.

References

1   Dressler G. Human Resource Management. Prentice-Hall of India, New Delhi; 2008.

2   Currie D. introduction to Human Resource Management: A Guide to Personnel in Practice. Pinnacle, New Delhi; 2006.

3   Sharma A, Khandekar A. Strategic Human Resource Management-An Indian Perspective. Response Books, New Delhi; 2006.

4   Fallon LF, Jr. and McConnell CR. Human Resource Management in Healthcare-Principles and Practice. Massachusetts: Jones and Bartlett Publishers, Inc.; 2007.

5   Francis CM et al. Hospital Administration. 3rd Ed. New Delhi: Jaypee Brothers Medical Publishers (P) Ltd; 2004: 124-37.

6   Goel S, Gupta AK, Singh A. Hospital Administration: A Problem Solving Approach. Reed Elsevier India Private Limited. 2014.

- Dr.Nilanjana, Dr.Arti Gupta, Dr.V.Reddy, Dr.Dipanjan Bandyopadhyay, Dr.Vidisha, Dr.Wasim, Dr.Sumit, Dr.Nabanita, Dr. Tanusree, Dr. Jarina had no changes
- Dr.Indranil had changes in the affiliation only
- Major changes by Dr. Rashmi, Dr.Sanjeev sir, Dr. Siddharth Mishra, Dr. P.Satpathy, Dr.Niraj, Dr. Rabbanie, Dr.Chandrashekhar, Dr, Satabd has been incorporated in the above compiled edits

CHAPTER 17

Health care policy and regulation

Dr Chandrasekhar Vallepalli

Assistant Professor, Department of Community Medicine,

SVIMS Sri Padmavathi Medical College for Women, Tirupati, Andhra Pradesh

Health Care Policy And Regulation

1. INTRODUCTION

Health care

Healthcare is the maintenance or improvement of health via the diagnosis, treatment, and prevention of disease, illness, injury, and other physical and mental impairments in human beings. Health care is delivered by health professionals in medicine, dentistry, midwifery, nursing, pharmacy, physical therapy, psychology and other allied health professionals. Health care is a basic human need. Individuals need clinical intervention to treat their injuries and illnesses, and communities benefit from the promotion of basic health and disease prevention practices. Health care covers not only medical care, but also all aspects of preventive health care.

Health Policy

The World Health Organization (WHO) defines Health policy as the "decisions, plans, and actions that are undertaken to achieve specific healthcare goals within a society». According to the World Health Organization, an explicit health policy can achieve several things: it defines a vision for the future; it outlines priorities and the expected roles of different groups; and it builds consensus and informs people.

Healthcare policy

The establishment and implementation of laws, rules, and regulations for administering the nation's healthcare system is referred to as healthcare policy. The healthcare system consists of services provided by medical professionals to diagnose, treat, and prevent mental and physical illness and injury.

Regulation

Regulation plays an important role in the healthcare industry. Various regulatory organisations safeguard the public against a variety of health risks and offer a variety of public health and welfare services. These regulatory entities work together to preserve and regulate public health at all levels.

2. Need For Health Care Policy

With the increasing Indian population over the recent decades, with changing demographics and social economy, and with the economy expanding at a rate of more than 7%., there have been significant changes in the healthcare requirements of the country. Over the years, Indian Healthcare system has made significant progress in various health indicators, such as life expectancy and maternal and child mortality. The government has rolled out several policies and undertaken missions both in rural and urban areas.

The major objectives of the health care policy are:

- To promote the health through preventive, promotive and curative intervention to the community.
- To provide affordable health care services to the community.
- To provide standardization in daily operational activities.
- It helps in setting a general plan of action used to guide desired outcomes and is a fundamental guideline to help make decisions.
- To set the foundation for the delivery of safe and cost effective quality care.
- To help prevent the spread of infections or diseases, provide education for healthier choices and practices, ensure health safety, and improve the overall quality of life for the public.

3. Different Types of Health Policies

Health policy can be divided into different types, each of which involves different components of health care. Some important examples include:

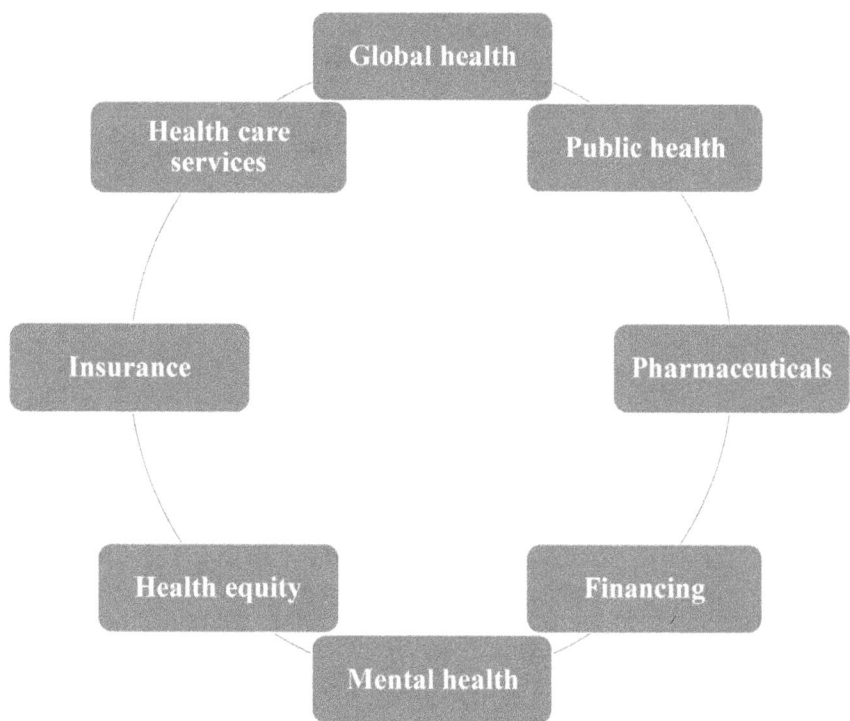

Figure 1: Different types of health policies

1. Global health: Global health offers a broad picture approach, assessing the health needs of people all around the world and striving for equity of care.

2. Public health: Public health describes policies enacted at the national, state, or community level to promote healthy lifestyles and prevent the spread of infectious diseases.

3. Pharmaceuticals: Pharmaceutical products regulation, availability and affordability may be addressed in the health policy.

4. Financing: Health policy may determine how to provide funding for medical services, including the extent to which the state reimburses for services from health facilities.

5. Mental health: Mental health care is an important factor when developing health policy, as it establishes goals and objectives for promoting mental well-being and treating those who suffer from mental illnesses.

6. Health equity: The stated goal of many health policies is to ensure that care is provided fairly in different communities and demographics.

7. Insurance: Health policies may also determine the role of insurance in financing care, promote affordable or public insurance options, and regulate what insurance companies can and cannot do.

8. Health care services: The compilation of health policies will directly affect the types of health care services available in a region.

4. National Health Care Policies

The Indian government enacts a number of acts and legislation which pertain to medical profession and education, nursing profession and education, pharmacists and pharmacy education, dental profession and education, mental health, drugs standards, advertisements relating to drugs and medicines, prevention of the extension from one State to another of infectious or contagious diseases affecting human beings and prevention of adulteration of foods and drugs to promote healthy lives for all. The government of India has rolled out various health care policies related to health care which are given in Table 1.

Table 1: National Health care policies in India

National Health Policy	Year
National Policy for Rare Diseases	2021
National Health Profile	2019
National Patient Safety Implementation Framework	2018
National Health Policy	2017
National Youth Policy	2015
National Mental Health Policy	2014
Home Based New Born Care Operational Guidelines	2014
India Newborn Action Plan (INAP)	2014
Kangaroo Mother Care & Optimal Feeding of Low Birth Weight Infants	2014
National Policy for Access to Plasma-derived Medicinal Products from Human Plasma for Clinical/ Therapeutic use	2014
National Urban Health Mission (NUHM)	2013

National Health Policy	Year
National Policy for Children	2013
National Charter for Children	2013
National Pharmaceutical Pricing Policy	2012
National Water Policy	2012
National Health Research Policy	2011
National Vaccine Policy	2011
Right of children to Free and Compulsory Education Bill—2009 (education to children aged between 6 and 14 years)	2009
National Blood Policy	2007
National Environment Policy	2006
National Policy for Persons with Disabilities	2006
National Rural Health Mission (NRHM)	2005
National charter for children	2003
National Youth Policy	2003
National Health Policy	2002
National Blood Policy	2002
National Policy on Indian System of Medicine and Homeopathy	2002
National Policy for Empowerment of Women	2001
National Population Policy	2000
National Policy on Older Persons	1999
National Nutrition Policy	1993
National AIDS Control and Prevention Policy	1992
National Health Policy	1983

5. Health Care Regulations

Table 2.1: Important regulations related to health care

Regulation	Year
The National Commission for Allied and Healthcare Professions Act	2021
Indian Medical Council (Professional Conduct, Etiquette and Ethics) (Amendment) Regulations	2020
The Consumer Protection Act	2019
The National Medical Commission Act	2019
Surrogacy (Regulation) Act	2018
Food Safety and Standards (Contaminants, Toxins and Residues) Regulations	2011

Regulation	Year
Food Safety and Standards (Prohibition And Restrictions On Sales) Regulations	2011
Food Safety and Standards (Laboratory and Sample Analysis) Regulations	2011
The Clinical Establishments (Registration and Regulation) Act	2010
The Prohibition Of Sexual Harassment Of Women At Workplace Bill	2010
The Marriage Laws (Amendment) Bill	2010
The Transplantation of Human Organ Rules	2008
The Food Safety and Standards Act	2006
The Protection of Women from Domestic Violence Act	2005
The Cigarettes and other Tobacco Products (Prohibition of trade, commerce, production, supply and distribution) Act	2003
The Indian Medical Council Act, 1956 (Professional conduct & Ethics) Regulations	2002
National Trust for Welfare of Persons with Autism, Cerebral Palsy, Mental Retardation and Multiple Disabilities Act	1999
Persons with Disabilities Rules	1996
Persons with Disabilities (Equal Opportunities, Protection of Rights and Full Participation) Act	1995
The Transplantation of Human Organs Rules	1995
The Transplantation of Human Organs Act	1994
the Rehabilitation Council of India Act	1992
The Mental Health Act	1987
The Narcotic Drugs and Psychotropic Substances Act	1985
The Homeopathy Central Council Act	1973
Insecticides Rules	1971
The Indian Medicine Central Council Act	1970
Registration of Births and Deaths Act	1969
Insecticides Act	1968
The Prevention of Food Adulteration Act	1954
The Dentists Act	1948
The Pharmacy Act	1948
The Indian Nursing Council Act	1947
The Drugs and Cosmetics Act	1940
The Red Cross Society (Allocation of Property) Act	1936
The Societies Registration Act	1860
The Epidemics Disease Act	1897

Table 2.2: Various regulations related to women and child health

Regulation	Year
Medical Termination of Pregnancy (Amendment) Act	2021
Medical Termination of Pregnancy Rules	2003
The Prenatal Diagnostic Techniques (Regulation and Prevention of misuse) Rules	1996
The Prenatal Diagnostic Techniques (Regulation and Prevention of misuse) Act	1994
Pre-conception and Pre-natal Diagnostic Techniques (Prohibition of Sex Selection) Act	1994
The Infant Milk Substitutes, Feeding Bottlers and Infant Foods (Regulation of Production, Supply and Distribution) Act	1992
The Juvenile Justice Act	1986
The Child Labor (Prohibition and Regulation) Act	1986
Family Court Act	1984
Medical Termination of Pregnancy Act	1971
The Maternity Benefit Act	1961
The Dowry Prohibition Act	1961
The Immoral Traffic (Prevention) Act	1956
The Child Marriage Restraint Act	1929

Table 2.3: Regulations for the protection of workers and their families and the legislations related to Environment

Regulation	Year
Legislations for protection of workers and their families	
The Rights of Persons with Disability Act	2016
The Sexual Harassment of Women at Workplace (Prevention, Prohibition and Redressal) Act (PoSH Act)	2013
The Child Labour (Prohibition and Regulation) Act	1986
The Dock Workers (Safety, Health and Welfare) Act	1986
The Dangerous Machine (Regulation) Act	1983
The Cine Workers Welfare Fund Act	1981
The Bonded Labor System (Abolition) Act	1976
The Equal Remuneration Act	1976
The Bidi Workers Welfare Fund Act	1976
The Mines Labor Welfare Fund Act	1972
The Contract Labor (Regulation and Abolition) Act	1970

Regulation	Year
The Beedi and Cigar Workers (Conditions of Employment) Act	1966
The Mines Act	1952
The Employees' Provident Fund and Miscellaneous Provisions Act	1952
The Plantation Labor Act	1951
The Factories Act	1948
The Employees State Insurance (ESI) Act	1948
The Minimum Wages Act	1948
The Industrial Disputes (ID) Act	1947
The Trade Union Act	1926
The Workmen's Compensation Act	1923
Environmental legislations	
Bio-Medical Waste Management (Amendment) Rules	2018
Compensatory Afforestation Fund (CAMPA) Act	2016
The Noise Pollution (Regulation and control) (Amendment) Rules	2010
The Biological Diversity Act	2002
The Motor Vehicles Act	1988
The Environment (Protection) Act	1986
The Air (Prevention and Control of Pollution) Act	1981
The Forest (Conservation) Act	1980
The Water (Prevention and Control of Pollution) Act	1974
The Wildlife Protection Act	1972
Prevention of Cruelty to Animals Act	1960
The Atomic Energy Act	1962
Wild Life (Protection) Act	1942
The Indian Forest Act	1927
Destructive Insect and Pest Act	1914

6. Constitutional Health Care Provisions

Some of the relevant constitutional provisions related to health care were:

1. **Article 21:** No person shall be deprived of his life or personal liberty except according to a procedure established by law.
2. **Article 23:** Prohibits and criminalises human trafficking and forced labour.
3. **Article 24:** Prohibition against the employment of children under the age of 14 in factories, mines and other dangerous work.

4. **Article 25:** The right to an adequate standard of living.

5. **Article 32:** Right to Constitutional Remedies. It allows all the Indian citizens to move to the country's Apex Court in case of violation of Fundamental Rights.

6. **Article 39:** Children are given opportunities and facilities to develop in a healthy manner and in conditions of freedom and dignity and that childhood and youth are protected against exploitation and against moral and material abandonment.

7. **Article 41:** The State shall within the limits of its economic capacity and development, make effective provision for securing the right to work, to education and to public assistance in cases of unemployment, old age, sickness and disablement, and in other cases of undeserved want.

8. **Article 42:** Provision for just and humane conditions of work and maternity relief.

9. **Article 47:** The State shall endeavour to bring about prohibition of intoxicating drinks and drugs that are injurious to health.

10. **Article 51:** The State shall promote international peace and security by the prescription of open, just and honourable relations between nations.

7. National Health Policy

After the National Health Policy 1983 commenced by the Parliament of India and updated in 2002 which served well in guiding the approach for the health sector in the Five-year plans, the Union Government approved the National Health Policy in 2017 which was aimed to cover the bottom 50% (500 million people) of the country's population working in the unorganized sector.

The primary aim of the National Health Policy, 2017, is to inform, clarify, strengthen and prioritize the role of the Government in shaping health systems in all its dimensions- investments in health, organization of healthcare services, prevention of diseases and promotion of good health through cross sectoral actions, access to technologies, developing human resources, encouraging medical pluralism, building knowledge base, developing better financial protection strategies, strengthening regulation and health assurance.

Key Policy Principles includes Professionalism, Integrity and Ethics; Equity; Affordability; Universality; Patient Centered and Quality of Care; Accountability; Inclusive Partnerships; Pluralism; Decentralization and Dynamism and Adaptiveness.

The policy identifies coordinated action on seven priority areas for improving the environment for health:

1. The Swachh Bharat Abhiyan
2. Balanced, healthy diets and regular exercises.
3. Addressing tobacco, alcohol and substance abuse
4. Yatri Suraksha – preventing deaths due to rail and road traffic accidents
5. Nirbhaya Nari – action against gender violence
6. Reduced stress and improved safety in the work place
7. Reducing indoor and outdoor air pollution

The policy also articulates the need for the development of strategies and institutional mechanisms in each of these seven areas, to create Swasth Nagrik Abhiyan – a social movement for health. It recommends setting indicators, their targets as also mechanisms for achievement in each of these areas.

8. Summary:

The final target of these wide frameworks of policies, programmes, acts and legislations are with providing good health and wellbeing to all the people in the community. The diverse challenges pose threat to achieving targets. Health care policies should be planned for making a robust preventive healthcare system which is an optimal solution to ease down the pressure building on the current healthcare system. Preventive healthcare in terms of proper sanitation, timely vaccination, avoidance of self-medication, increasing awareness through health education and regular health check-ups should be promoted through government policies. The government should pay more attention to implementation, not just promoting such programs. Healthcare policies and regulations are essential in providing clarity when dealing with issues and activities that are critical to the health and safety, legal liabilities and regulatory requirements. We need solution driven healthcare policies and regulations to the challenges which are best suited to our community and our systems. Appropriate policy action will determine the future direction of the healthcare sector in India.

References

1. Srinivisan R. Health care in India – Vision 2020: Issues and Prospects [Internet]. Niti.gov.in. [cited 25 January 2021]. Available from: https://www.niti.gov.in/planning commission.gov.in/docs/reports/genrep/bkpap2020/26_bg2020.pdf

2. WHO. National health policies, strategies, plans [Internet]. Who.int. [cited 25 January 2021]. Available from: https://www.who.int/nationalpolicies/nationalpolicies/en/

3. What is Health Policy? [Internet]. University of North Dakota Online. [cited 25 January 2021]. Available from: https://onlinedegrees.und.edu/blog/what-is-health-policy/

4. Garg S. Healthcare Policy in India- Challenges and Remedies [Internet]. Iima.ac.in. [cited 10 March 2021]. Available from: https://www.iima.ac.in/c/document_library/

   Shivani%20Garg_Public%20Policy_Healthcare0ea5.pdf?uuid=f4758624-d359-4608-82e7-abb73ad2f51f&groupId=52123

5. Grover A, Singh R. Health Policy, Programmes and Initiatives. Advances in Geographical and Environmental Sciences. 2019; 251-266.

6. Acts. Ministry of Health and Family Welfare. GOI [Internet]. Main.mohfw.gov.in. [cited 30 March 2021]. Available from: https://main.mohfw.gov.in/acts-rules-and-standards-health-sector/acts

7. Kishore J. Legislation and health promotion in India. DRUNPP Rev Global Med Healthcare Res. 2012; 3(2):75–87.

8. Rao K, Panchamukhi P. Health and the Indian Constitution. CMDR Monograph Series No. - 7 [Internet]. Cmdr.ac.in. [cited 20 March 2021]. Available from: http://www.cmdr.ac.in/editor_v51/assets/Mono-7.pdf

9. National Health Policy 2017. Ministry of Health and Family Welfare. GOI [Internet]. Nhp.gov.in. 2017 [cited 25 January 2021]. Available from: https://www.nhp.gov.in/nhpfiles/national_health_policy_2017.pdf

Chapter 18

Evaluation of Ongoing Health Programmes

Dr. Abhilash Sood,

Professor and Head Department of Community Medicine
Dr. Radhakrishnan Government Medical College Hamirpur Himachal Pradesh

Dr. Mitasha Singh,

Assistant Professor, Department of Community Medicine
ESIC Medical College Faridabad Haryana

Evaluation: A Successor of Monitoring or a Synonym?

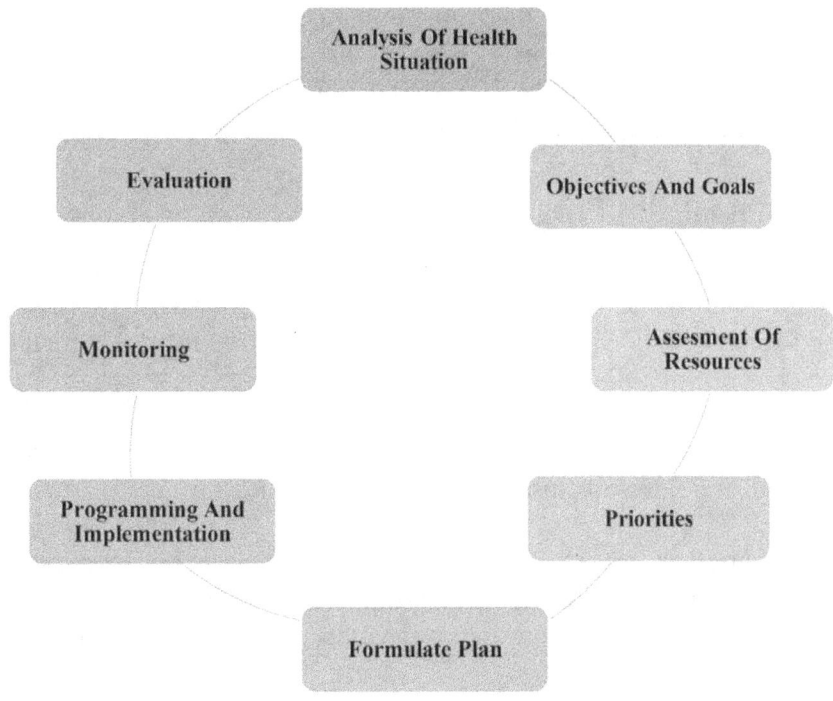

Planning Cycle in Health

The planning cycle is used in any situation, event or ongoing activities of health system management. One of the most important and probably the last step in planning is evaluation. With every evaluation a new plan is prepared. "To evaluate" is simply defined as to judge the value of. Generally, the term evaluation is used to include the whole process of examination or measurement and the ultimate judgment of value. [1]

Monitoring is a planned process of observation that closely follows a course of activities, and compares what is happening with what is expected to happen. Monitoring requires periodic collection and review of information on programme implementation, coverage and use for comparison with implementation plans, identifies shortcomings, provides elements of analysis as to why progress fell short of expectations, modifying original plans during implementation if required. It is a day-to-day activity during implementation of a programme.

Evaluation always follows monitoring. It measures the quality of a health programme. It is a systematic process to determine the extent to which service needs and results have been or are being achieved and analyse the reasons for any discrepancy. It is an attempt to measure service's relevance, efficiency and effectiveness.

Table 1: Comparing Monitoring and Evaluation

	Monitoring	Evaluation
Focus on	Input and output	Outcome and impacts
Process	Collecting data on progress	Assessing data at critical stage of process
Periodicity	Continuous	Periodic
Utilisation	Alerts managers to problems	Provides managers with strategy and policy options

Input in terms of national health programmes denotes the manpower, resources and time put in the programme at the implementation stage. Outputs are the programme services received by the population it is intended to deliver. Outcomes are depicted by the change in population/client behaviour or skills receiving the programme. The improvement in health status of population is the impact of the programme. Output, outcome and impact are the dependent variables of a programme which are measured using Monitoring and Evaluation.

Why Evaluate National Health Programmes?

National health programmes aim to prevent or control disease, injury, disability and death. Health programmes address problems of large numbers of community members and organisations. Unlike the previous century, where vaccination and sanitation solved major problems, current times involve difficult changes in attitudes and risk/protective behaviour of population.

Moreover, programmes that perform well in some settings fail miserably in others because of the socioeconomic, demographic, interpersonal, and inter-organisational settings in which they are planted.

Data gathered during evaluation enables managers and staff to create the best possible programmes, to learn from mistakes, to make modifications as needed, to monitor progress toward program goals, and to judge the success of the program in achieving its short-term, intermediate, and long-term outcomes.

General Approach In Evaluation

Evaluation can be undertaken at different times and in various ways, but it follows certain general principles. The general approach in evaluation is as follows:

- Measurement of observed achievements
- Comparison with previously stated norms, standards or intended results
- Analysis of cause of failure
- Decision (feedback) [1]

Every evaluation uses a tool called Indicator. An indicator is a standardised, objective measure that allows a measure of the progress toward achieving programme goals, a comparison among health facilities, a comparison among countries, a comparison between different time periods.

Planning the Evaluation

Every health programme has a clear objective and goals to be achieved in a time bound manner. Hence, it is essential that the evaluation framework is developed and implemented alongside the proposed programme. It usually involves collecting data, in a baseline study, to assess the situation before going on to develop the programme.

The evaluation focuses on assessing the extent to which the programme objectives have been met, and may have one or more aims. Evaluation questions may be:

- Descriptive, where the aim is to observe, describe and measure changes
- Causal, where the aim is to understand and assess relations of cause and effect
- Performance-related, where evaluation criteria are applied
- Predictive, where an attempt is made to anticipate what will happen as a result of planned interventions
- Probing, where the intention is to support change, often from a value committed stance[2]

Types of Evaluation

Evaluation of national health programmes can be carried out in reference to impact or outcome, process and structure. The evaluation questions depend on how long the programme has been in existence, who is asking the question, and why the evaluation information is needed. The following types of evaluation have been further elaborated:

1. **Process/ Implementation Evaluation:** Evaluation of process examines whether the programme was carried out as planned. It measures the actual programme performance against the initial plan. This involves creating a list of indicators that need to be measured, depending on the aims of the programme. For example, in the Universal Immunization programme for infants and children in a village of India, a process evaluation may have following indicators:

(a) Proportion of facilities that maintained temperature records

(b) Proportion of facilities with complete stock registers

(c) Proportion of health facilities having an up to date coverage/drop-out monitoring charts

(d) Proportion of health workers counselling and giving key important messages

(e) Proportion of health workers giving PCM in DPT vaccines

(f) Proportion of AEFIs/ VPDs reported and investigated

The results help to identify the strengths and weaknesses of the programme, and where improvements may be made. This is also known as formative evaluation.

2. **Impact Evaluation:** This seeks a behaviour change in target population that has been brought about by the programme and which may have not occurred if the programme had not happened. It usually looks upon long term effects of programme.

3. **Outcome Evaluation:** Outcome denotes the success or failure of programme in terms of change in morbidity, mortality, quality of life, functional status, including symptom recognition and patient satisfaction. An example in terms of indicator for outcome evaluation of immunisation programme is change in infant mortality rate and incidence of vaccine preventable diseases. This is the most common form of evaluation.

Outcome is also measured by the health team's effectiveness, or achievement of results, performance of activities and efficiency, or economic use of resources.

Management Decisions Concerned with Outcome Evaluation Effectiveness Evaluation

It measures the results obtained by a programme as per its predetermined objectives. This is actually judging the value of results achieved by the health team. The information obtained is used to improve the quantity, quality, accessibility, efficiency, of services. Two questions must be asked by the evaluator: firstly, whether the results are those that were intended, and secondly, whether they are of value.

The general approach to evaluation consists of five steps:

* Deciding what aspects of programme are to be evaluated and how effectiveness is to measured
* Collecting information needed to provide the evidence
* Comparing the results with targets and objectives
* Judging whether and to what extent the targets and objectives have been met
* Deciding whether to continue the programme unchanged, to change it or to stop it

An example of effectiveness evaluation is as follows:

In a district of India, target of reducing the incidence of neonatal tetanus in 20 villages at the end of year X will be reduced to 1 per 1,000 live births from present (year Y) incidence of 5 per 1,000. For achieving this target of a programme, the following measurements are needed; (a) the yearly incidence (i.e. number of cases) of neonatal tetanus per 1,000 live births, (b) the rate at which the incidence falls from one year to another; and (c) the distribution of new cases among 20 villages. These three variables are direct measures of effectiveness of the programme. Ideally, baseline information (e.g., yearly incidence and the distribution of neonatal tetanus before target is set) should be obtained. Every case of neonatal tetanus must be reported to the evaluators at regular intervals. Usually, one person from each village (e.g., health volunteer) is responsible for recording and reporting the same at the end of every three-month period. The information obtained must be compared with the targets set for that period or time and for each place. Once comparisons were made the evaluation group must judge the value to the community of what has been achieved. Hence, in simple words, one must judge whether the annual and total incidence of neonatal tetanus has been reduced to the targeted figure, and whether the distribution norm has been met (e.g., no more than one case in each village) has been met. When results fall below what was expected, the reasons must be explored and analysed. Further decisions are to be arrived at if achievement is not satisfactory.

Efficiency Evaluation

It measures the output per unit of input. Work progress of a health team is evaluated to find out whether the team completed the work that was assigned to it in order to reach its targets (quantity), whether the work was of the expected quality and was carried out on time, and whether the budget was overspent or not. Evaluation for efficiency follows same five steps as effectiveness evaluation.

Continuing with the previous example of neonatal tetanus; to control it, in the district, three critical activities are needed. These are: (a) trained birth attendants (TBA) to be retrained in sterile handling of umbilical cord (a developmental activity); (b) mothers to be immunised at antenatal clinics (a service activity); (c) messages on prevention of neonatal tetanus to be spread to people (a support activity). The information on retraining TBAs may be measured as the number trained per month or number who have passed some qualifying test. Immunised mothers may be expressed as a number or as a percentage of pregnant women in each village. Message spread may be measured at the source (newspaper, radio, etc.) at the receiving end (individual mothers reached) or at some intermediate point (village heads transmitting the information). Achievement may be compared with norms and targets and expressed as rates or ratios. While analysing the information, various instances may come up. For instance, it is found that in some villages, training of TBAs and spread of messages by village heads are up to expectation (targeted level), but immunization coverage is far below the district average. Here, the relation between three activities in other villages needs to be studied. The results should be judged on the basis of a clear understanding of local situation. Further, the conclusions are communicated to decision makers who control the programme. It may be decided at this stage whether performance must be further assessed or programme needs to be improved.

Performance Evaluation

It is done for the staff to improve or maintain satisfactory levels. The staff appraisal process also follows the same five steps. It should be emphasised to the appraiser and to the staff member whose performance is to be appraised, that it is not intended to find fault with staff, even when results fall short of what was intended. The indicators of performance appraisal are job description, a work plan and technical procedure manuals. In the previous example, the performance appraisal of nurse in charge of controlling neonatal tetanus in a district may be done against the results achieved, services delivered, TBAs retrained and messages reaching the community. This task is performed by management and not by the staff member. The comparison with norms must be carefully interpreted. Success in one area must be balanced against failure in another.

Cost/Economic Evaluation

It is concerned with how the resources used relate to results achieved over a period of, say, one year, with the aim of answering the following question: Could some resources achieve better results or outputs or could results be achieved with fewer resources. The process of evaluation follows the same five steps as above. A full economic evaluation can be undertaken using either of four designs: Cost Minimisation Analysis, Cost Effectiveness Analysis, Cost Utility Analysis and Cost Benefit Analysis.

Cost Minimisation Analysis compares the costs of two or more competing interventions, having common outcome measures and which have been found to be "equally effective". The cheapest one is the preferred alternative. For a cost-minimisation analysis to be a valid and reliable source of evidence to decision makers, it requires the availability of high-quality clinical evidence that proves the equivalence of two treatments its application.

Cost Effectiveness Analysis (CEA) compares the costs and outcomes of two or more alternatives or compares a new intervention or treatment with the status quo. Different interventions are measured using a single outcome; usually in "natural" units designed to capture the improvement in health status. Health outcomes could be measured as more distal indicator such as actual improvement in health (for example, life-years gained, deaths avoided), or a more proximal or intermediate outcome such as a clinical indicator resulting from the program (e.g., reduction in cholesterol levels). It relates the net costs associated with net health outcome, such as cost per disease avoided, cost per death avoided, or cost per additional expected life year. The net cost includes the cost of delivering a specific health intervention to prevent a disease or unwanted health outcome minus the treatment and other costs not incurred because of the beneficial effects of the intervention. The value of this incremental cost effectiveness ratio (ICER) implies that the programme 'X', as compared to program 'Y', costs an additional Rs ABC per death prevented or disease prevented or life year gained.

Using cost effectiveness analysis with independent programmes requires that cost effectiveness ratios (CERs) are calculated for each programme and placed in rank order.

CER = Costs of intervention

Health effects produced (e.g., life years gained)

Cost-effectiveness of Three Independent Programmes

Programme	Cost (INR)	Health Effect (Life Years Gained)	CER
Z	1,50,000	1,850	81.08
Y	1,00,000	1,200	83.33
X	1,20,000	1,350	88.89

For example, in Table 2, there are three interventions for different patient groups, with the alternative for each of them of "doing nothing". According to cost-effectiveness analysis, programme Z should be given priority over X since it has a lower CER, i.e., for per unit of benefit achieved the programme 'Z' costs least. In order to decide which programme/ programmes to implement, the extent of resources available or the budget constraint must be considered. This implies that we can continue to prioritise in terms of programme 'Z', followed by 'X', and lastly 'Y'. If the budget required exhausts after implementing programmes Z and X, then Y will not be considered for implementation.

Cost Utility Analysis (CUA) employs utility-based measures to assess benefits. "Utility" is a term used by economists to refer to the subjective level of wellbeing that people experience in different health states. In simple words, "utility" as used by economists refers to happiness or pleasure. It incorporates the dimension of quality of life into the measurement of benefits. Benefits are measured as "quality-adjusted life-years," or QALYs, in which the gain in expected lifespan resulting from an intervention is weighted by the quality of that life, as assessed through some type of systematic survey of the affected (or general) population.

Cost Benefit Analysis (CBA) is an evaluation method in which the benefits of the health intervention are expressed in monetary terms. In so doing, benefits from a health care programme become commensurable with the benefits from any other public (or private) sector programme. CBA is broader in scope (as opposed to CEA and CUA which address mainly questions of technical efficiency) and can answer questions of allocative efficiency because it assigns relative values to health and non- health related goals in determining which goals are worthwhile. CBA compares the discounted future streams of incremental programme benefits with incremental programme costs. The difference between the two streams is the net social benefit of the programme; a positive net social benefit indicating that a programme is worthwhile. However, placing a rupee value on health benefits is an exercise fraught with conceptual and empirical difficulties. The sensitivity of the CBA result to assumptions about the value of life renders the method of limited practical value in the field of health policy. [3, 4]

Use of Epidemiology to Evaluate Health Services

In health services, research independent variable in focus is the health service, with reduction in adverse health effects as the anticipated outcome (dependent variable) if modality of care is effective. On the other hand, the etiological epidemiologic research the possible relationship between a cause (independent variable) and an adverse health effect or effects (dependent variable) is examined. Hence, most of the study designs used in etiological studies are common to health services research.

Ecologic Studies: Two indices can be used in ecologic studies. Avoidable mortality which analyses rate of avoidable death should vary inversely with the availability, accessibility, and quality of medical care in different geographic regions. This will serve as a measure of adequacy and effectiveness of care in an area. However, data on confounders may not be available and the resulting inferences may therefore be open to question. Another index is use of health indicator like incidence of certain conditions.

Randomised Design: The study participants are assigned to receive one type of care versus another rather than to receive care versus no care.

Non Randomised designs: Not all interventions and programmes can be subjected to randomised trials. The most common reason is of logistic complexities and the expenses involved. Also, ethical problems are perceived to occur in health services in evaluation studies. Randomised trials take long time to complete because healthcare programmes and health problems change over time. Hence, many researchers use data from non-randomised studies that often use large existing data sets.

Before After Design: Another study design to evaluate a programme is to compare people who received care before a programme was established with those who received care from the programme after it was established. The problem with this design is that the data obtained in each of the two periods are frequently not comparable in terms of either quality or completeness. The data on people treated after the new program begins may be collected using a well-designed research instrument, whereas data for past patients may include only that which may be available from healthcare records that had been designed and used only for clinical or administrative purposes. The difference in outcome observed may or may not be due to effect of programme or due to some other factors that may have changed over time like housing, nutrition, socioeconomic status, or use of other health services. Another disadvantage is that it is difficult to know whether the population studied after a programme was established is actually similar to that seen before the programme was established in terms of other factors that might affect outcome.

Hence, before after design provide a suggestion and are rarely conclusive in demonstrating the effectiveness of a new health service.

Non Randomised Designs (Programme no Programme): To avoid changes over time, another design could be a simultaneous comparison of two populations that are not randomised, in which one population is served by the programme and the other is not. This type of design is a cohort study in which the type of health care being studied represents the "exposure." As in any cohort study, the problem arises as to how to select exposed and unexposed groups for study.

Comparison of Utilisers and Non-utilisers: This design compares a group of people who a health service with a group of people who do not. To address selection bias, the prognostic profile of those who use care and those who do not can be characterised. Further improvement can be done by using eligible and non-eligible population. Eligibility or non-eligibility is not related to either prognosis or outcome; therefore, no selection bias is being introduced that might affect the inferences from the study. Eligibility criteria may include the type of employer or the census tract of residence. Ineligible persons can be selected from similar neighborhoods that could compensate for the concern with ensuring comparability of socioeconomic status. In addition, as differences between eligible and ineligible individuals may also affect external validity, on occasion adjustment for the variables that differ between these individuals improves external validity.

Combination Designs: One can combine a before–after design with a programme–no programme design or eligible ineligible design.

Case Control Designs: The evaluation of vaccines and other forms of prevention and screening programs can be done by use of the case-control design. It is primarily used for etiologic designs but can also serve as a surrogate for randomised trials. The "exposure" is then the specific preventive or other health measure that is being assessed. As in most health services research, stratification by disease severity and by other possible prognostic factors is essential for appropriate interpretation of the findings.

Observational Design: These include time series analysis, cross sectional surveys, and case studies. Case studies may be particularly appropriate for assessing changes in public health capacity in disparate population groups, different settings, when a unique outcome is being. [5]

Data Collection Sources

After deciding upon the objectives, indicators and design of evaluation next step will be identifying data collection methods and sources. These can be existing data sources (secondary data collection) or new data will be collected (primary data). Depending on your evaluation questions and indicators, some secondary data sources may be appropriate. These can be:

- Census of country
- National family health survey (NFHS) reports

- District level health survey (DLHS) reports
- Health management information system (HMIS) records for every district and village
- Cancer registries
- Integrated diseases surveillance programme databases
- Other disease registries

Primary data collection methods are

- Surveys, including personal interviews, telephone interviews and instruments completed by responder
- Group discussions
- Observations
- Document review (medical records, minutes of meetings, logs an diaries)
- Key informants

The context and content of objective must be considered before choosing the right method from the many secondary and primary data collection choices. *Context* denotes: How much money can be devoted to collection and measurement? How soon are results needed? Are there ethical considerations? *Content* means: Is it a sensitive issue? Is it about a behaviour that is observable? Is it something the respondent is likely to know?) [3, 6]

Analysis and Synthesis of Data

The collected data is systematically tabulated, summarised and compared with other appropriate information to extract useful information that responds to the evaluation questions. Interpretation is the effort of determining what the findings mean, making sense of the evidence gathered in an evaluation and its practical applications for effectiveness.

References

1. R McMohan, E Barton, and M Piot. 'On Being in Charge: A Guide to Management in Primary Health Care'. *World Health Organization*, 2nd ed. India: AITBS publisher, 2007.
2. World Health Organization. 'WHO Evaluation Practice Handbook'. Geneva: WHO Press, 2013.
3. ME Drummond, GL Stoddard, and GW Torrance. *Methods for the Economic Evaluation of Health Care Programmes*, 1st ed. Oxford University Press, 1987.
4. BJ O' Brien. *Principles of Economic Evaluations for Health Care Programs*, 22: pp 1399-1402. J Rheumatol, 1995.
5. L Gordis. *Epidemiology*, 5th ed. Canada: Elsevier, 2014.
6. U.S. Department of Health and Human Services Centers for Disease Control and Prevention. Office of the Director, Office of Strategy and Innovation. 'Introduction to Program Evaluation for Public Health Programs: A Self-study Guide'. Atlanta, GA: Centers for Disease Control and Prevention, 2011.

Chapter 19

Newer Advents in a Pandemic: Evolution of Drugs viz. Evolution of HAART During HIV/AIDS

Dr Dipanjan Bandyopadhyay

Professor and Head of the Department, Dept of Medicine,

North Bengal Medical College, West Bengal

BACKGROUND

The pandemic of HIV/AIDS continues to devastate people and nations. However, with rapid and meaningful strides coming in the domain of antiretroviral therapy, HIV has transformed itself from a uniformly fatal illness to a chronic, manageable disease. Spectacular discoveries and unprecedented philanthropy combined to bring about this change in our lifetimes. This article is a tribute to the glorious panorama of antiretroviral therapy.

From Monotherapy to HAART

In 1987, the first antiretroviral agent, zidovudine (AZT), a nucleoside reverse transcriptase inhibitor (NRTI), was shown to have a positive impact on clinical progression and death. This was a time of unforeseen optimism and premature jubilation, apparently heralding the victory over the virus. However, the challenges of early NRTI regimens were soon evident. These included high pill burdens, inconvenient dosing, treatment-limiting toxicities and incomplete virological suppression. Inadequate virological suppression resulted in the emergence of multiple resistance mutations, with long-term treatment consequences. Protease inhibitors (PIs) and non-nucleoside reverse transcriptase inhibitors (NNRTIs), introduced in the mid-1990s, revolutionized the management of HIV infection. A triple drug combination therapy), consisting of two NRTIs (Stavudine, Zidovudine, Abacavir, Didanosine, Zalcitabine or Tenofovir which is a nucleotide reverse transcriptase inhibitor, NtRTI) plus a PI or NNRTI, was capable of effective and durable virological suppression. The widespread use of these combinations rapidly led to dramatic reductions in morbidity and mortality in the developed world. The strategy of using two NRTIs plus a potent third agent still forms the cornerstone of current treatment principles, and is now referred to as highly active or combination antiretroviral therapy (HAART or cART). Combination of three (or more) anti-HIV compounds is aimed at the same goals as for the treatment of tuberculosis: (a) to obtain synergism between different compounds acting at different molecular targets; (b) to lower the individual drug dosages to reduce their toxic side effects; and (c) to diminish the likelihood of development of drug resistance.

Drug Adversities and Regiment Durability

HAART itself was not devoid of difficulties. High pill burdens, inconvenient dosing, stringent food requirements, treatment-limiting toxicities and numerous drug interactions attenuated the success of HAART. Moreover, unrealistic levels of adherence (≥95 per cent) were required to maintain adequate ART exposure and sustain viral suppression. Drug related toxicities abounded and initial experience with the thymidine analogs, d4T (Stavudine) and AZT (Zidovudine) led to disfiguring lipoatrophy. Protease inhibitors were limited by unfavourable pharmacokinetic (PK) characteristics, including limited oral bioavailability, short half-lives, significant inter- and intra-patient variability, propensity for drug interactions, risk of resistance, toxicity and storage/stability issues. The NNRTIs (Nevirapine, Efavirenz) had the advantage of long half-lives, but disadvantages of toxicities, drug interactions and single mutation conferring high level class resistance. The search continued for a better HAART.

When to Start

The timing of HAART had remained a matter of controversy until recent years. Initial guidelines recommended HAART only at CD4 counts below 200, which moved to 250 and thereafter to 350 over the course of the past two decades. The SMART (Strategies for Management of Antiretroviral Therapy) study, which randomised patients either to continuous therapy or a drug-conservation arm, with either planned deferral of initial therapy until CD4 <250 cells/mm³ or CD4 count — guided discontinuation of treatment. The study unequivocally proved that those patients randomized to drug conservation had significantly more morbidity and mortality in comparison to those on continuous therapy, and put to rest the notion of 'drug holidays' as a viable solution to pill fatigue and toxicities. More recently, the Strategic Timing of Antiretroviral Therapy (START) trial was published in 2015 and established the current concept that early initiation of HAART irrespective of the CD4 count or clinical condition reduces long term mortality and morbidity. This was further strengthened by the HIV Prevention Trials Network (HPTN) 052 trial which showed that antiretroviral therapy (ART) prevented more than 96 per cent of genetically linked infections caused by human immunodeficiency virus type 1 (HIV-1) in sero-discordant couples, and thus emerged the concept of treatment as prevention (TasP). This also established a strong case for the early initiation of HAART. Today, upfront HAART at the time of HIV detection is uniformly advocated across all guidelines.

FDC

With PIs becoming the state of the art at the turn of the millennium, they needed to be dosed three times daily, either fasting or with a significant meal and/or liquid intake, amounting to impractical daily pill burdens. Moreover, they were associated with significant metabolic consequences in the form of dyslipidemia, dysglycemia, osteoporosis and renal stones. In 2006, the approval of co-formulated tenofovir/FTC/efavirenz allowed for the first "one pill, once a day" regimen. Several fixed-dose combination products are now available which augments adherence and therapeutic success.

Pharmaco-enhancement

A significant advance in treatment was achieved with the concept of pharmaco-enhancement with Ritonavir. The demonstration that low-dose ritonavir (100–200 mg daily) could be used to increase the systemic bioavailability of the accompanying cytochrome P450 3A4 substrate PI was a major advance. The addition of Ritonavir as a pharmaco-enhancer allowed simplification to once or twice daily administration and led to improved patient adherence and virological outcomes, particularly in treatment experienced patients, where boosted regimens had the ability to overcome low-level PI resistance. A new pharmacokinetic enhancer, cobicistat, is now available to inhibit the CYP3A enzyme without antiretroviral activity. At a dose of 150 mg, it was found to exhibit similar CYP3A4 activity to Ritonavir 100 mg. This led us to the quad pill which contains tenofovir difumarate (TDF) and emtricitabine (FTC), in addition to cobicistat (COBI; an inactivator of cytochrome P450 isoenzyme CYP3A without anti-HIV activity) and a new integrase inhibitor, elvitegravir (EVG). The quad does not have drug interactions with H2-receptor antagonists or proton pump inhibitors, does not cause central nervous system (CNS) side effects, and is pregnancy category B.

Integrase Strand Transfer Inhibitors (INSTI)

Coming to the birth of newer drug classes, the traditional NRTI, NNRTI and PIs continue to serve as faithful members of the growing ARV hierarchy. Although integrase has been pursued for many years as a potential target for the development of new anti-HIV compounds, the first integrase inhibitor (INSTI) Raltegravir was approved in 2007. This was followed by Elvitegravir and Dolutegravir (DTG). DTG is a drug that is more effective, easier to take and has fewer side effects than alternative drugs that are currently used. DTG also has a high genetic barrier to developing drug resistance, which is important given the rising trend of resistance to efavirenz and nevirapine-based regimens. Based on new evidence assessing benefits and risks, the WHO in 2019 recommended the use of DTG as the preferred first-line and second-line treatment for all populations, including pregnant women and those of childbearing potential.

Further Drugs

Among other drug classes, fusion inhibitors and co-receptor inhibitors have made an entry into the market. Enfuviritide is the lone fusion inhibitor (FI) currently available for the treatment of HIV infections. It must be administered subcutaneously twice daily, thus compromising its use in population settings. Co-receptor inhibitors (CRIs) interact with the co-receptors CCR5 or CXCR4 used by M (macrophage)-tropic or R5 and T (lymphocyte)-tropic or X4 HIV strains respectively to enter the target cells. The CCR5 antagonist maraviroc was licensed in 2007 but is only active against R5 HIV strains. When used on a mixed population of X4/R5 HIV strains, they stimulate the selection of X4 strains. Ideally, a CCR5 antagonist should be combined with a CXCR4 antagonist so as to block both X4 and R5 HIV strains.

TAF (Tenofovir Alafenamide) is a prodrug. In the body, TAF is converted to tenofovir diphosphate (TFV-DP). TAF is designed to circulate systemically as the prodrug and undergo conversion to tenofovir intracellularly, achieving higher active metabolite concentrations in peripheral blood mononuclear cells and lower plasma tenofovir exposures than Tenofovir Disoproxil Fumarate (TDF) does. Replacing TDF with TAF is routinely practiced by nowadays, reducing nephrotoxicity of TDF.

Biologics as HAART

Ibalizumab is the first monoclonal antibody to be approved for the treatment of HIV-1 infection. As a CD4-directed post-attachment inhibitor, ibalizumab blocks HIV-1 entry into CD4 cells while preserving normal immune function. Ibalizumab, in combination with other antiretroviral(s), is indicated in the USA for the treatment of heavily treatment-experienced adults with multidrug-resistant HIV-1 infection failing their current antiretroviral regimen, and in the EU for the treatment of adults infected with multidrug-resistant HIV-1 infection for whom it is otherwise not possible to construct a suppressive antiviral regimen.

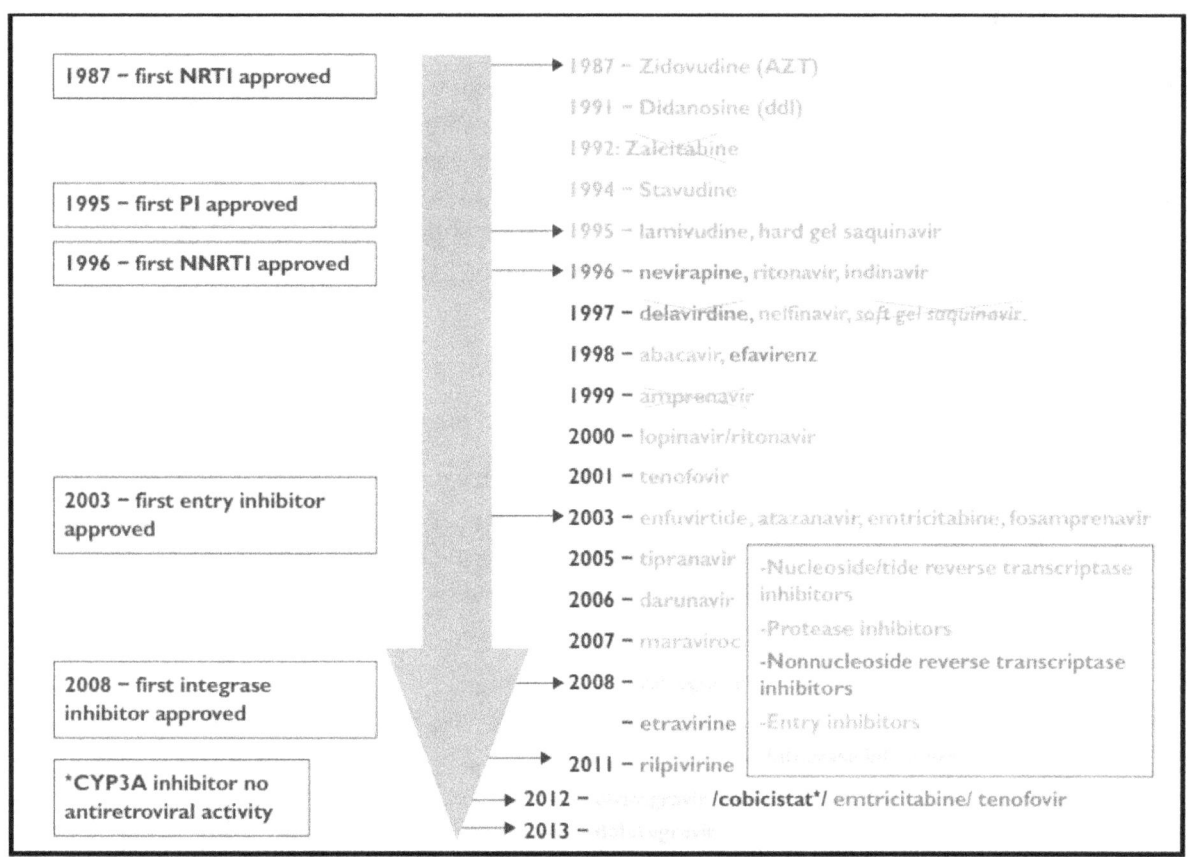

Figure 1: The time course of development ART drugs, highlighted according to the US Food and Drug Administration (FDA) approval date. Those that are no longer in use or available are illustrated with an 'X' through them

Table 1: Currently available antiretroviral drugs

Nucleoside Reverse Transcriptase Inhibitors (NsRTI)	Non Nucleoside Reverse Transcriptase Inhibitors (NNRTI)	Protease Inhibitors (PI)
• Zidovudine (AZT/ZDV)	• Nevirapine (NVP)	• Saquinavir (SQV)
• Stavudine (d4T)	• Efavirenz (EFV)	• Ritonavir (RTV)
• Lamivudine (3TC)	• Delavirdine (DLV)	• Nelfinavir (NFV)
• Abacavir (ABC)	• Rilpivirine (RPV)	• Amprenavir (APV)
• Didanosine (ddl)	• Etravirine (ETV)	• Indinavir (INV)
• Zalcitabine (ddC)	**Integrase Inhibitors**	• Lopinavir (LPV)
• Emtricitabine (FTC)	• Raltegravir (RGV)	• Fosamprenavir (FPV)
Nucleotide Reverse Transcriptase Inhibitors (NtRTI)	• Elvitegravir (EVG)	• Atazanavir (ATV)
	• Dolutegravir (DTG)	• Tipranavir (TPV)
• Tenofovir (TDF)		• Darunavir (DRV)
Fusion Inhibitors (FI)	**CCR5 Entry Inhibitor**	**Monoclonal Antibody**
• Enfuvirtide (T 20)	• Maraviroc	• Ibalizumab

ART beyond HAART

Post exposure prophylaxis (PEP) for HIV has always depended upon ART. Tenofovir 300 mg + Lamivudine 300 mg + Efavirenz 600 mg once daily for 28 days has been the standard regimen for PEP in India, although PI based PEP is now advocated. The strategy of using antiretroviral therapy in individuals at high risk of acquiring HIV (i.e., pre-exposure prophylaxis or PrEP) represents another significant milestone in HIV therapeutics. In 2012, Tenofovir/Emtricitabine became the first regimen to receive an FDA indication for PrEP. Above all, the prevention of parent to child transmission (PPTCT) has been one of the most glorious successes of antiretroviral therapy.

Emerging Technologies

The future is busy for antiretroviral drugs. Nanotechnology to develop long-acting injections of antiretroviral drugs is being explored. Current injectable nano-formulations that are under study include the second-generation NNRTI Rilpivirine and a new long-acting integrase inhibitor (GSK-1265744). GSK-1265744, a dolutegravir analogue, is detectable in plasma up to 48 weeks following a single injection.

Where We Stand

The story of antiretroviral drugs has unfolded in many unexpected domains. From the concept of mono-therapy with a single agent, we now consider mega HAART and giga HAART which might include five or seven drugs in a regimen. Furthermore, newer drugs have emerged, making life simple and effective for the patient and the provider alike. Last, treatment as prevention (TasP) has become a reality. Currently, out of the 2.3 million PLHIV in India, 76 per cent know their HIV status, among those 84 per cent are on treatment, and among the PLHIV on treatment whose viral load is measured 84 per cent are virally suppressed.

The Government of India launched "Test and Treat" model on 28 April 2017 to put PLHIV on ART as soon as they are detected HIV positive, irrespective of their CD4 count. The objective was to improve the survival rate and quality of life of HIV infected persons at the individual level. In 2019-20, for every 100 HIV infected people identified at HIV counseling and testing centers, 88 PLHIV were initiated on ART. Recent decisions to roll-out more efficacious treatment regimens [Dolutegravir] and multi-month dispensation to ensure further expanded treatment coverage and retention will further reduce AIDS-related deaths and HIV transmission in the country. The emergence of durable regimens which might be administered intermittently shall actually halt the spread of this epidemic and possibly lead us to the dream of cure. Till then, it is a story of evolution.

Further Readings:

1. ED Clercq. 'Anti-HIV drugs: 25 Compounds Approved Within 25 years After the Discovery of HIV'. *International Journal of Antimicrobial Agents*, 33: pp 307–320. 2009.
2. MS Saag, CA Benson, RT Gandhi, JF Hoy, RJ Landovitz, MJ Mugavero, et al. 'Antiretroviral Drugs for Treatment and Prevention of HIV Infection in Adults 2018: Recommendations of the International Antiviral Society–USA Panel'. *JAMA*, 320(4): pp 379-96. 2018.

3. KA Vaidya, AV Kadam, and V Nema. 'Anti-Retroviral Drugs for HIV: Old and New'. *Austin J HIV/AIDS Res,* 3(2): p 1026. 2016.

4. K Maedaa, D Das, T Kobayakawa, H Tamamura, and H Takeuchi. 'Discovery and Development of Anti-HIV Therapeutic Agents: Progress Towards Improved HIV Medication'. *Current Topics in Medicinal Chemistry 2019,* 19: pp 1-29.

5. A Tseng, J Seet, and EJ Phillips. 'The Evolution of Three Decades of Antiretroviral Therapy: Challenges, Triumphs and the Promise of the Future'. *Br J Clin Pharmacol* 79; 2: pp 182–194.

6. National AIDS Control Organization. 'Sankalak: Status of National AIDS Response', 2nd ed. New Delhi: NACO, Ministry of Health and Family Welfare, Government of India, 2020.

Chapter 20

New Set Ups in the Pandemic: Challenges, Barriers and Way Forward

Dr Nilanjana Ghosh

Assistant Professor, Dept of Community and Family Medicine,

All India Institute of Medical Sciences, Guwahati

COVID 19 was a unique public health challenge that we faced, and it was also the most dreaded one. After an initial furore and mayhem, after the chaos and catastrophe, came the lull before the storm: the planet came to a standstill. By the time it had prepared to face the wrath, widespread disaster and destruction had already occurred. Cold statistics revealed some frightening data and before one knew it, the entire world had gone into a lockdown. Healthcare workers faced their toll of staying away from their families, wearing PPE suits and also, at times, working without them. Every health institution formed teams at various levels and tried to combat the crisis in the best possible way. Regular, routine OPDs had stopped by a point of time[1].

Soon, COVID 19 screening clinics, institutional quarantine centres and isolation wards were opened to screen, detect and treat patients who were COVID positive. It was a big thing even a year back, but now rampant positive cases have diluted the fear. However, the stigma related to COVID is yet to take a backseat. Testing kiosks, VRDL laboratories, COVID vaccination clinics, well equipped COVID blocks with adequate HFNO and recently, COVID segregation clinics began to be opened. These were in addition to RICU, which is mainly for high density unit ICU patients; the latter deals with interdepartmental transit and were formed to combat the menace[1,2].

This is a brief overview of how tertiary medical colleges are run, specifically those located in the rural foothills of the Himalayan subterrain, coping with its own set of problems due to geographical location and consequent human resource availability. Dedicated staff, 24*7 supportive supervision from select seniors and college administration have played a pivotal role in changing these places to success stories, notwithstanding the challenges, barriers and limitations faced. It is assumed that in India, the three-tier public healthcare delivery care system works on relatively similar infrastructure and logistics.[3]

Usual Challenges That Need to be Faced and Resolved[2-4]

- Infrastructure, logistics, new and changing directives, initial hiccups. Designating hospitals in accordance with the new pandemic, like opening of SARI and COVID hospitals
- Challenges specific to the region need to be addressed. If far away from HQ, then there is strangulation of resource availability during national lockdown. Difficult terrains, harsh climates can be a problem

- Streamlining COVID management protocol and healthcare staff. Forming a rapid response time with healthcare workers willing to devote extra hours
- Human resource management – both availability and accessibility. Need stringent laws to enforce leave bans during crisis time because if any person tests positive, the shortage increases as the total pool of HCW is fixed
- Huge catering population as, with other routine healthcare systems stalled, neighbouring states also come for care. No refusal policy, and district coordination are an issue, as well as handling media, who add to the mayhem
- Reorientation of general masses attending health care facility, living around it, dealing with the dead, dealing with emergency patients, segregating suspects from those affected in case they get admitted/test positive after admission
- Lack of provision of special designated beds for HCWs
- Reporting and monitoring

Usual Barriers Encountered [1,3,5] –

- Difficulty in customising care as per the local health settings if directives are pan India/pan state as variegated geographical and epidemiological profiles exist with cultural diversity
- Funds and autonomy to serving medical colleges needs to be allotted. Human resource shortage needs to be addressed since, if hospitals refuse admission even overnight, a huge socio-political stir will be created
- Plight of serving HCWs needs to be addressed rather than portraying them as warriors/martyrs. Dealing with the mental health component of HCW and patient is necessary but often neglected
- Need for vaccination among family members of HCWs; this is as pertinent as vaccinating HCWs themselves
- Ever changing COVID protocols need to be percolated well, across all tiers of society. All nursing homes and private practitioners need to be united in the test, trace and treat policy. Laws can be helpful. A common protocol on treating the dead may be made
- Oxygen support in remote peripheries became a major problem as also the limited health facilities, restricted workforce availability and accessibility

Way Forward

Salutogenic perspectives are new indicators for good health. It is imperative than salutogenic model slowly takes over the pathogenic model just as the preventive behaviours have taken over. A concept of well-being supporting factors that enhance human health rather than those that focus on disease its primarily predicted by Sense of Coherence (SOC), Researchers correlated high SOC with a better health outcome than a person with low SOC given the same health condition[6]. These models have potential to usher sea change during COVID if appropriately applied. Its components are:

1. **Sense of Meaningfulness:** A belief that things in life are a source of satisfaction and that people have a purpose to carry out. Job participation, motivation, job congruence, job control and task significance all relate to this.
2. **Sense of Manageability:** Sense that have the resources and skill to keep things under control under any circumstances. This creates a sense of well-being. Mainly relates to social skills and trust.
3. **Sense of Comprehensibility:** A belief that things happen in orderly fashion and can be predicted. Mostly relates to consistent feedback at work and performance appraisals.

Hence, High SOC and Wellness can be Ensured by:

1. Reaching the hitherto unreached by initiating a bidirectional communication despite having limited access information technology. It will increase uptake of preventive behaviours preached once their queries are addressed and fears allayed[7].

2. Salutogenic perspectives during designing hospital infrastructure like COVID blocks and reorienting the existing ones. Health promoting hospitals with community engagement and keeping in mind ergonomics, occupational and safety management is the new key to enhanced health and increasing self-care ability of patients[8].

3. Addressing the neglected mental health component with support from Covid care NGOs who work in autonomy but in accordance with state governance — health being a state responsibility.

4. Monitoring and supervision from senior medical associations and implementing newer concepts like Jugaru OPD.

References

1. World Health Organization Department of Communications. 'Novel Coronavirus (2019-nCoV): Strategic Preparedness and Response Plan'. 2019. Available at: https://www.who.int/internal-publications-detail/updated-country-preparedness-and-response-status-for-covid-19-as-of-19-march-2020 [Google Scholar]

2. GRID COVID-19 Study Group. 'Combating the COVID-19 Pandemic in a Resource-constrained Setting: Insights from Initial Response in India'. *BMJ Global Health*. 2020; 5:e003416. doi:10.1136/bmjgh-2020-003416.

3. MZ Sadique, WJ Edmunds, RD Smith, WJ Meerding, O de Zwart, J Brug, et al. 'Precautionary Behavior in Response to Perceived Threat of Pandemic Influenza'. *Emerg Infect Dis*, 13(9): pp 1307–13. September 2007. Available at: http://www.cdc.gov/eid/content/13/9/1307.htm

4. Centers for Disease Control and Prevention. 'Implementation of Mitigation Strategies for Communities with Local COVID-19 Transmission'. 2020. https://www.cdc.gov/coronavirus/2019-ncov/downloads/community-mitigation-strategy.pdf

5. Y Alimohamadi, M Taghdir, and M Sepandi. 'The Estimate of the Basic Reproduction Number for Novel Coronavirus Disease (COVID-19): A Systematic Review and Meta-analysis'. Korean J Prev Med. 2020

6. S Bhattacharya, KB Pradhan, MA Bashar, S Tripathi, A Thiyagarajan, A Srivastava, and A Singh. 'Salutogenesis: A Bona Fide Guide Towards Health Preservation. *J Family Med Prim Care*, 9:16-9. 2020.

7. VL Champion, and CS Skinner. 'The Health Belief Model'. Health Behav Health Educ Theory Res Pract, 4: pp 45–65. 2008.

8. MB Mittelmark, S Sagy, M Eriksson, et al., eds. 'The Handbook of Salutogenesis'. *Application of Salutogenesis in Hospitals*, ch 27. Cham (CH): Springer, 2017. [last accessed on 25.5.2021]

Chapter 21

Community Resource Management

Dr Tanushree Mondal

Associate Professor, Dept of Community Medicine, Calcutta Medical College, Kolkata

Deputy Director of Medical Education, Swasthya Bhavan, West Bengal

Community Resource Management and Human Resource Management

In our day-to-day life, we adopt various strategies to make our life better, and easier. Though it seems an easy affair, it does require a whole lot of planning beforehand, so that we come out with the desired outcome. We, in fact, explore all those possibilities that can improve the quality of life of not only our family, but also the entire community at large. Therein comes the role of the so-called concept of the Community Resource Management (CRM), and therein lies the importance of CRM.

Definition

Community Resource Management is a process tailored to the needs and traditions of local groups, which aims to create equitable and sustained access to natural resources, while minimising damage to ecosystems on which they depend. CRM is also known as Community Based Natural Resource Management (CBNRM).

Human Resource Management, or HRM, is the practice of managing people to achieve better performance.

Differences Between CRM and HRM:

Characteristics	Community Resource Management	Human Resource Management
What it is:	Multi-stakeholder collaboration that involves all participants, from communities, to government, to NGOs, and promotes coordination among them	It is also known as personnel management. It is a specialised field that emphasises recruitment and management of people working for a certain organisation
What it deals with:	Conflict management mechanisms – support processes to manage natural resource conflicts among stakeholders	It deals with compensation, benefits, hiring, firing, safety, wellness as well as training of employees

Characteristics	Community Resource Management	Human Resource Management
What it includes:	Participatory action research – collaborative fact-finding and analysis generates a mutually agreed upon perspective for action	It involves planning, organising, directing, controlling of the performance of operative functions
What it constitutes:	Strong local organisations, such as forest-farmer groups and inter-village networks are built from the bottom-up	It constitutes application of management functions and principles, and integration of the decisions of the employees
What it embodies:	Livelihood improvement and environmental services. We work to sustain environmental conservation by linking it to farm and community enterprises. Provide opportunities for reinvestment by linking upland environmental services to lowland and urban communities	The scope of HRM extends to every strategy, factor, principles, operations, practices, functions, activities and methods related to management of employees
What it includes:	Policy support and law enforcement are essential to curbing illegal encroachment leading to ecosystem degradation	Objectives are varied

Example of CRM in the Present Scenario

Natural resource managers are increasingly being asked to work with diverse stakeholder groups and incorporate their values and objectives when developing conservation plans.

Such decisions are fraught with the complexity and uncertainty associated with ecological system dynamics and multiple and potentially conflicting objectives under consideration.

Here, we address these problems as "WICKED" problems just because there is a whole realm of social planning problems that cannot be successfully treated with traditional linear and analytical approaches. The terminology was originally proposed by HWJ Rittel and MM Webber, both urban planners at the University of California, Berkeley, USA in 1973. Such problems may be varied, like the air pollution in Delhi, relocating villages from a tiger reserve, mitigating climate change, crop damage by Nilgai or issues like cleaning the river Ganga. Such problems are often complex and need to be identified, followed by applying a framework called the wicked problem framework; this will help analyse the situation by synthesising from disciplines such as social sciences, economics, environmental ethics and environmental sciences.

For example, the issue of air pollution in Delhi has multi causal factors. In the case of mitigation of climate change, there is the issue of environment versus development factors and issues of sacrificing present growth for future benefits. Similarly, the issue of crop damage by Nilgai involves issues which are difficult to define and have ethical issues involved. So also, in the case pertaining to cleaning the river Ganga, there are various stakeholders involved like sewage discharge, religious values versus industrial sludge, etc.

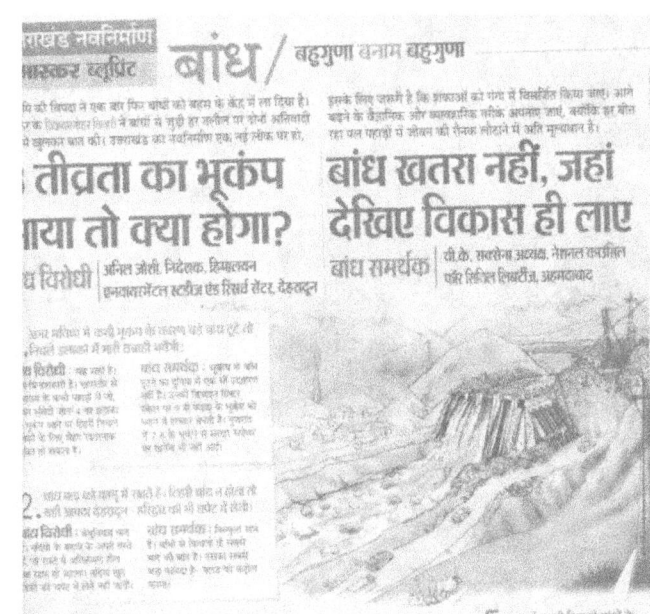

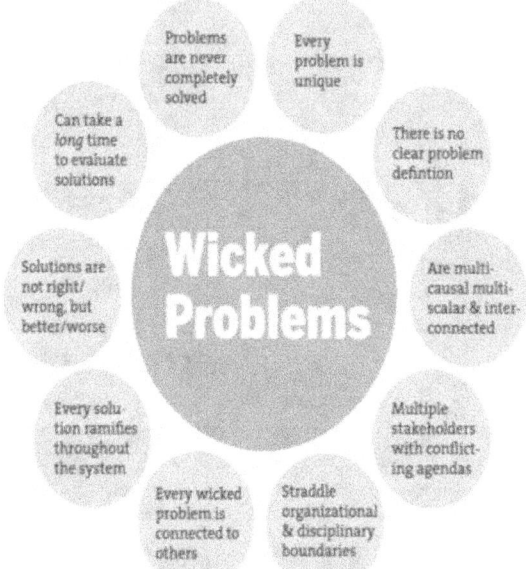

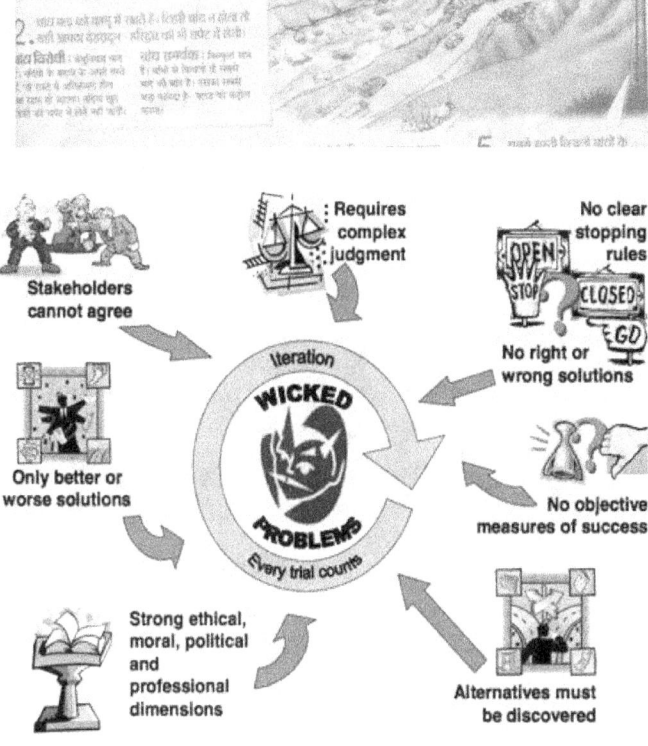

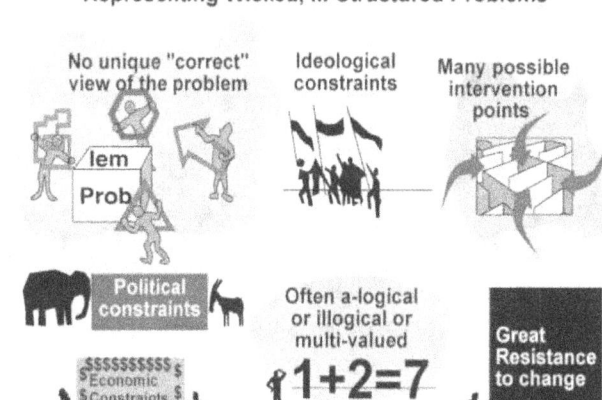

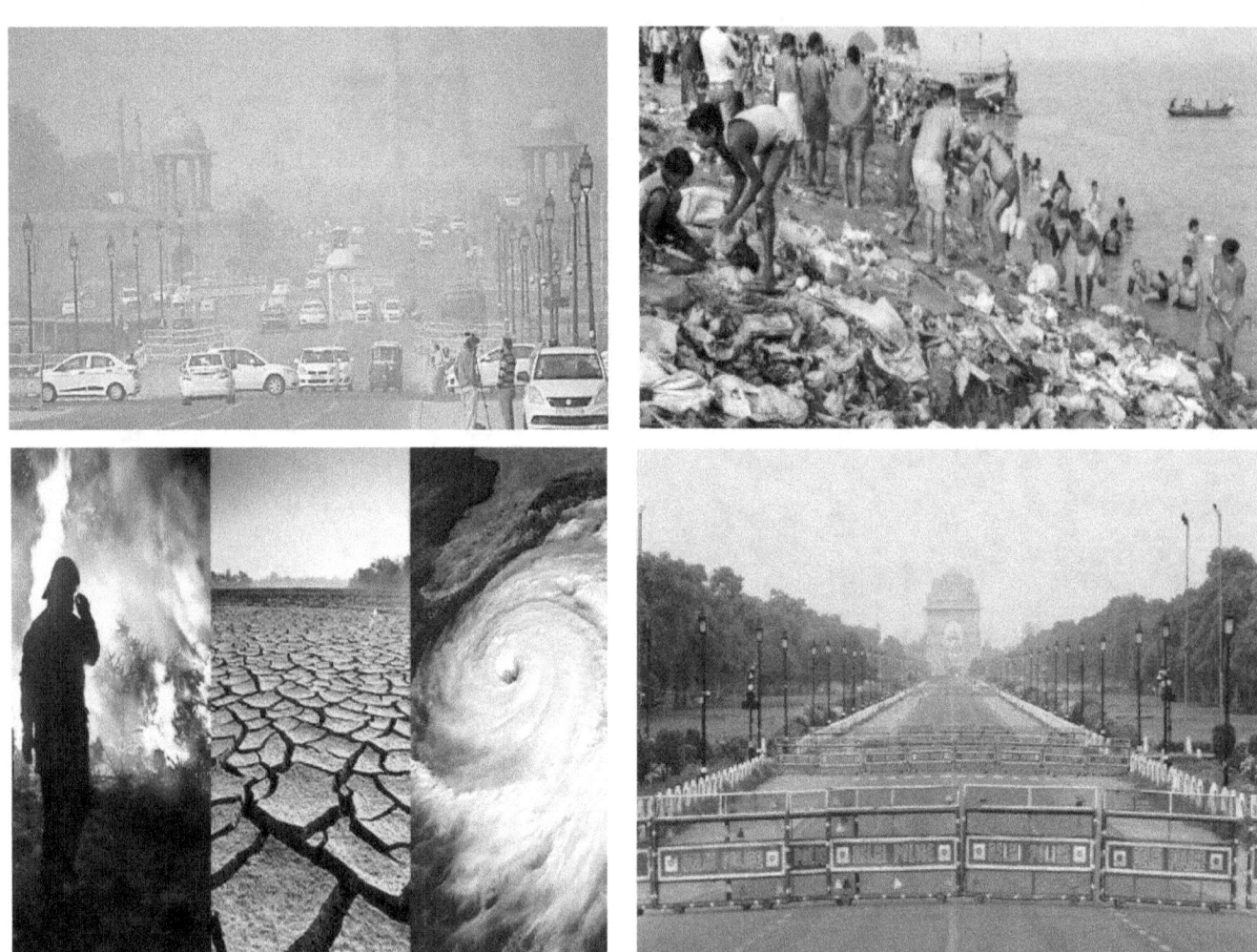

In tackling all the problems listed above, the possible solution may be involvement of science, political will as well as equitable sharing, collective action and leadership, and/or a combination of all of these factors.

Significance of CRM in the Present Context

Now is the era for maximising benefits out of the many resources available. As such, there lies a dynamic equilibrium between natural resource renewal and utilisation (water, soil, tress, local biodiversity) and CRM practically makes an attempt to monitor, supervise this equilibrium. It works for the establishment of such an equilibrium while sustaining the whole process, thereby aiming to alleviate problems like poverty, hunger, disease, famine, etc.

CRM is highly significant in today's world as it is a documentary of the community development, utilisation and the priorities for conservation in order to implement several resource management plans and activities and foreseeing the long-term benefits out of it.

CRM Process: In order to do an effective Community Resource Management, it is essential and prudent to have a CRM plan. This is actually an instrument or a tool for integrating the indigenous system of knowledge into the natural resource management proper.

The plan proper encompasses the various end points like:

1. Strategy
2. Desired state
3. Recommendations
4. Remarks

This whole process involves a multistakeholder collaboration with the government, NGOs, and CBOs, and engages them in conflict management mechanisms, participatory action research, network formation, livelihood improvement, law enforcement and policy decisions support mechanism, in addition to collaborative management plans.

Thus, CRM is the mantra of the near future if we have to live happily and sustain our existence on this beautiful planet.

References

1. https://www.wn.org/what-we-do/community-based-natural-resources-management/
2. https://www.researchgate.net/publication/277832605The_Community_Resource_Management_Plan:_A_Tool_for_Integrating_Indigenous_Knowledge_Systems_into_Natural_Resource_Management/figures'
3. https://www.wn.org/what-we-do/community-based-natural-resources-management/

Colored Images and Tables

CHAPTER 1

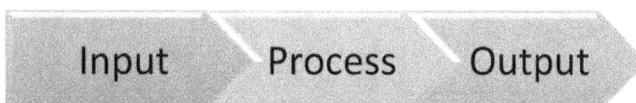

Figure 1: The steps of health management system

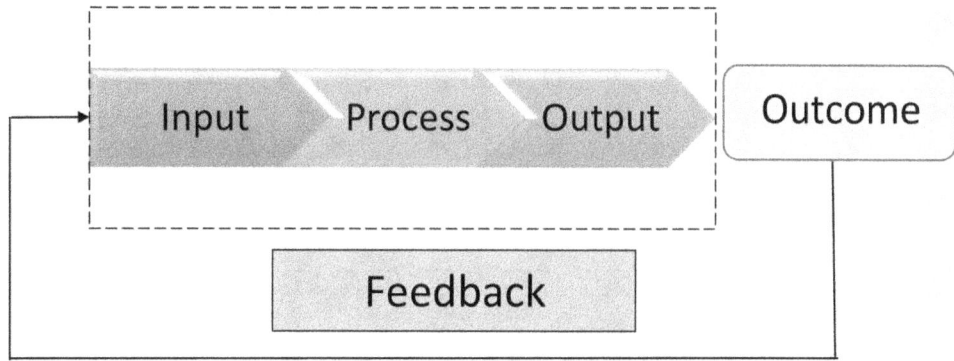

Figure 2: The steps of health management system with outcome and feedback

CHAPTER 2

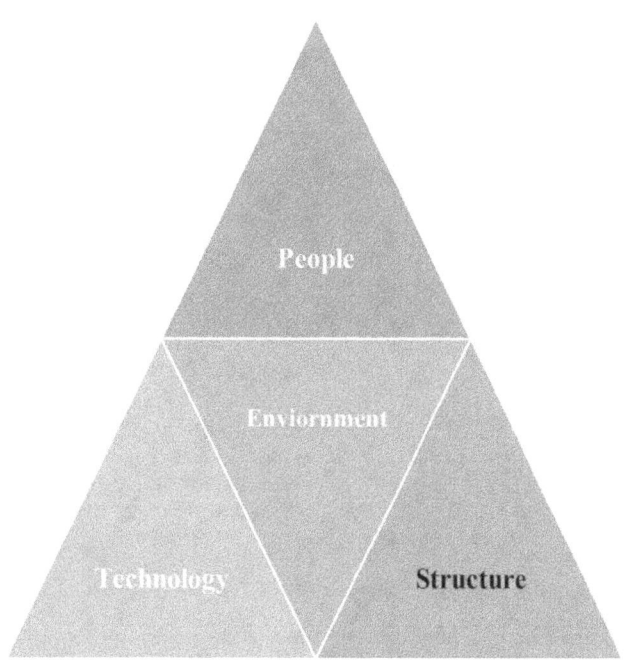

Brainstorming	1. Five and ten in number 2. Free association 3. Main focus is on generation of ideas and not on evaluation of these ideas 4. More ideas can be originated 5. Very effective when the problem is comparatively precise and simply defined
1. Similar to brainstorming except that this approach is more structured 2. Members do not communicate well with each other so that strong personality domination is evaded 3. Group coordinator either collects the written ideas or writes them on a large blackboard and discusses them 4. Highest cumulative ranking idea is selected as the final solution	**Nominal Group Thinking**
Didactic Interaction	1. Applicable only in certain situations 2. Type of problem should be such that it generates output in the form of yes or no
1. Improvised version of the nominal group technique 2. Opinions of experts physically distant from each other and unknown to each other 3. Process of sending questionnaires, results and review until we reach a final decision with agreement.	**Delphi Technique**

CHAPTER 4

Known to Self Known to Others **OPEN SELF**	Known to Self Unknown to Others **HIDDEN SELF**
Unknown to Self Known to Others **BLIND SELF**	Unknown to Self Unknown to Others **Undiscovered**

ABC	• *Always Better Control* • Annual consumption cost of items
VED	• *Vital, Essential, Desirable* • Vital and critical items
FSN	• *Fast moving, Slow moving and Non moving* • Issues from stores
SDE	• *Scare, Difficult, Easy* • Availability of items
HML	• *High, Medium and Low* • Unit price
XYZ	• Value analysis
SOS	• *Season Off Season* • Seasonal requirement

		V items		E items		D items			
	A Items	AV		AE		AD		Category 1 Items	
	B Items	BV		BE		BD		Category 2 Items	
	C Items	CV		CE		CD		Category 3 Items	

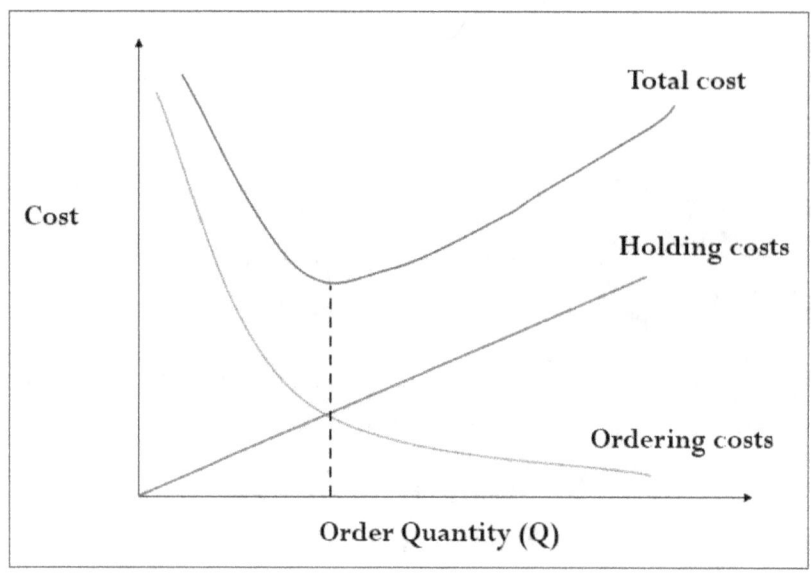

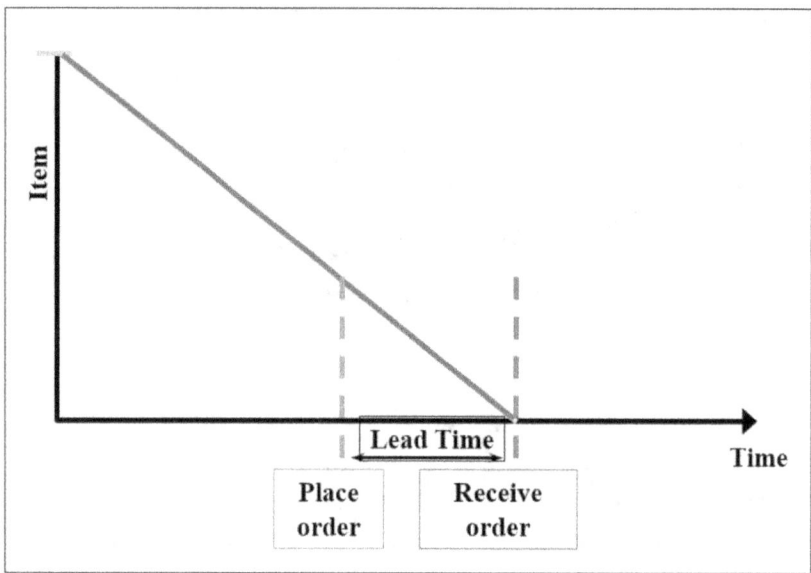

CHAPTER 6

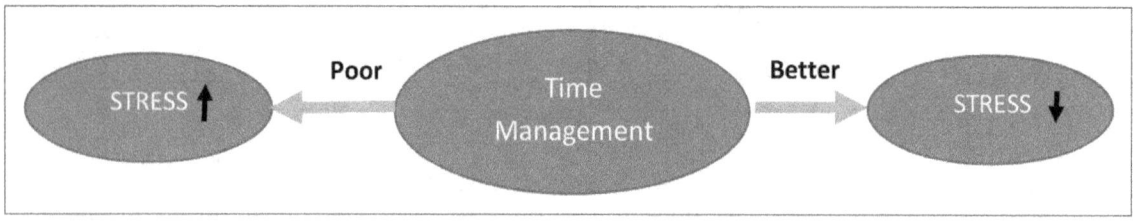

Fig.1: Relationship between time management and Stress

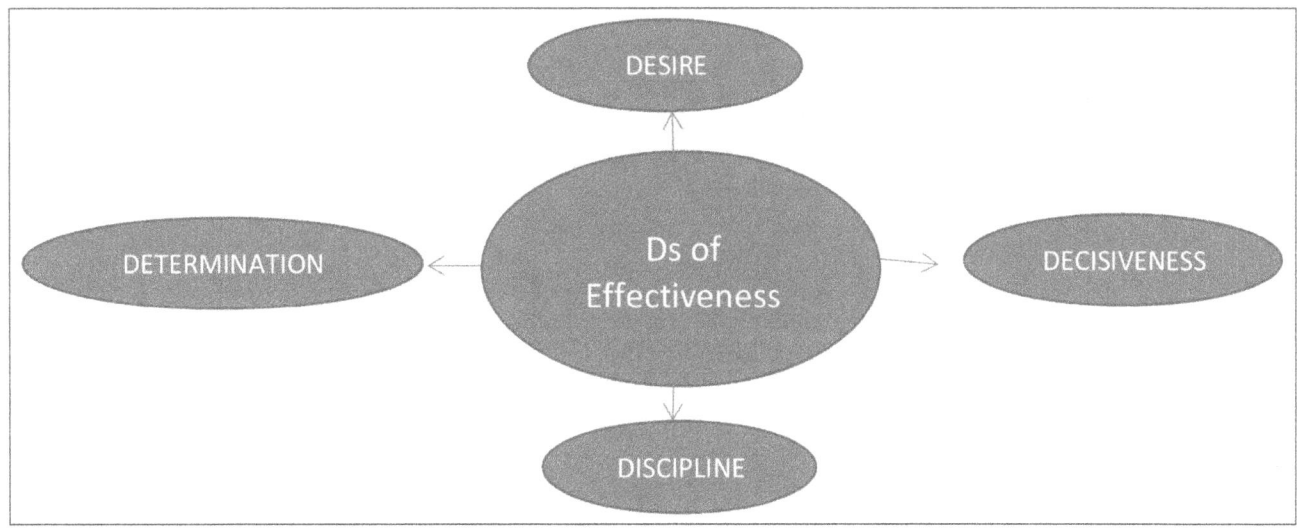

Fig 2. 4Ds of Effectiveness

CHAPTER 7

The term Management by Objectives was coined by Peter Drucker in 1954.

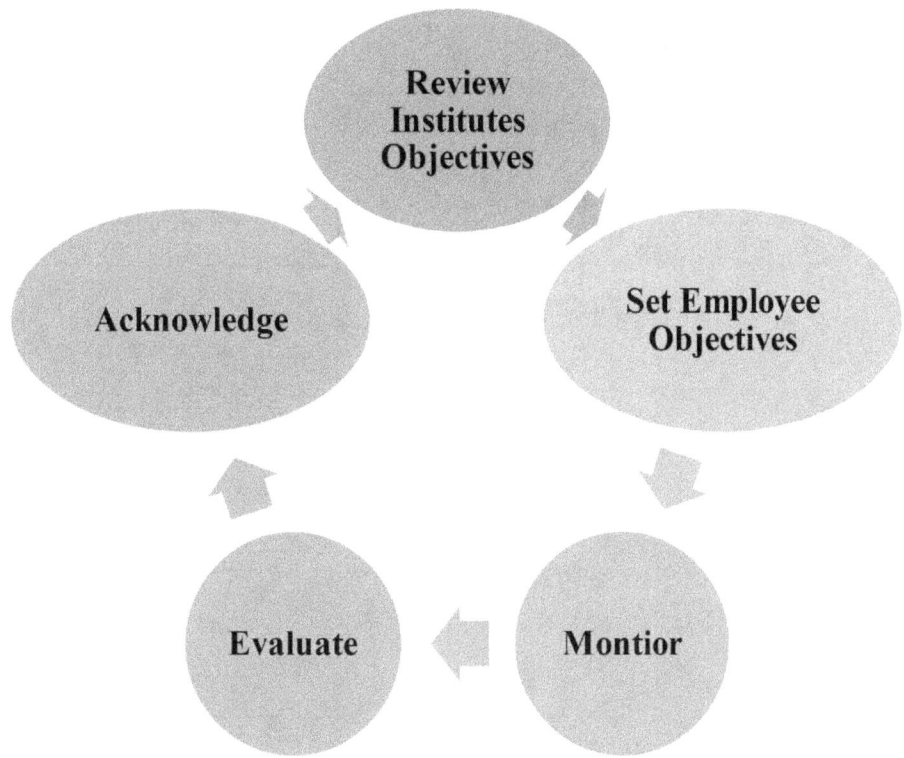

Chapter 10

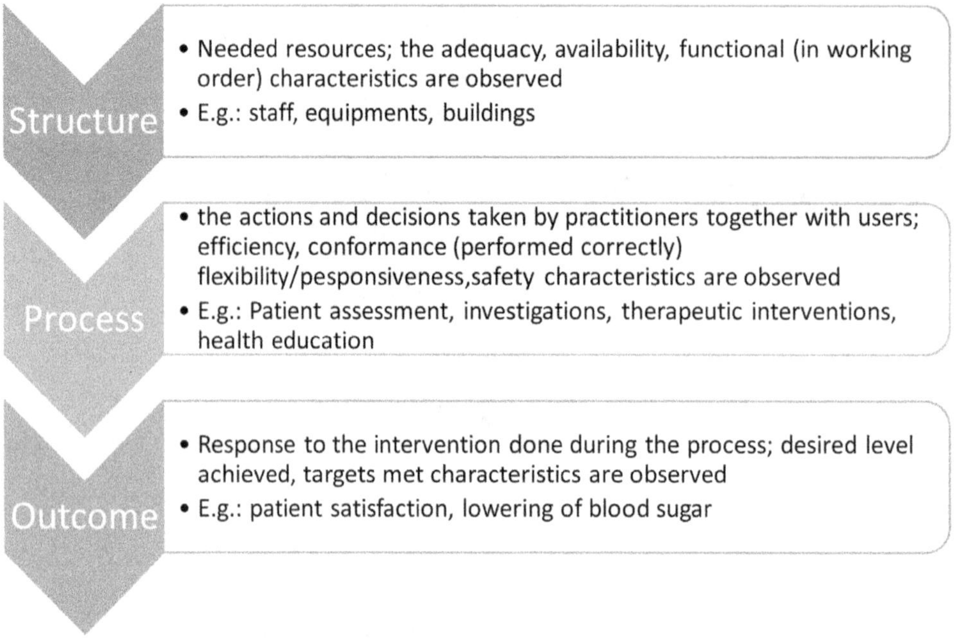

Structure
• Needed resources; the adequacy, availability, functional (in working order) characteristics are observed
• E.g.: staff, equipments, buildings
Process
• the actions and decisions taken by practitioners together with users; efficiency, conformance (performed correctly) flexibility/pesponsiveness,safety characteristics are observed
• E.g.: Patient assessment, investigations, therapeutic interventions, health education
Outcome
• Response to the intervention done during the process; desired level achieved, targets met characteristics are observed
• E.g.: patient satisfaction, lowering of blood sugar

Figure 2: Classification of Criteria

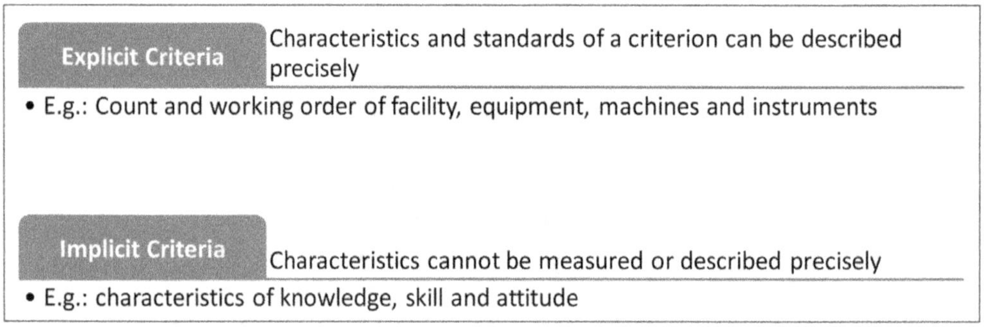

Explicit Criteria
Characteristics and standards of a criterion can be described precisely
• E.g.: Count and working order of facility, equipment, machines and instruments
Implicit Criteria
Characteristics cannot be measured or described precisely
• E.g.: characteristics of knowledge, skill and attitude

Figure 3: Explicit and Implicit Criteria

CHAPTER 12

Act
Plan
Study
Do
Act
Plan
Check
Do

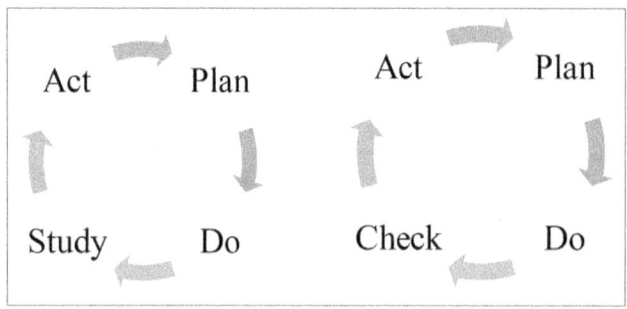

Figure 1: PDSA & PDCA Cycles

Table 2: Examples of indicators across domains of structure, process and outcome

Structure (or Input) Indicators	Process Indicators	Outcome indicators
❖ physical facility – space, number of beds, number of OTs, types of OTs, proximity to modes of transport etc ❖ interdepartmental relationship of functional units (eg presence of committee and board such as condemnation committee or tumour board etc) ❖ human resources – qualification, expertise & experience, job description, job content, job analysis at each position, knowledge & skill required, recruitment policy, human resource development policy, trainings (orientation/ongoing), defined & written duty/responsibilities of staff, supervision policy & guidelines etc ❖ staffing norms, selection criteria, selection process ❖ equipment with appropriate technology, purchase committee, purchase system, installation & maintenance programme, periodic validation, repair facilities, operation manuals, training ❖ materials (medicines, surgical items, dietary supplies etc) - demand assessment, specifications, drug formulary, drug selection committee, purchase committees, purchasing system, procedures on receipt/inspection//storage/issue, store management etc	❖ medical care ❖ nursing care ❖ supportive & utility care ❖ process evaluation through medical/nursing audit or peer review or death review or tissue review,medical records committee, utilization committee, hospital infection control committee, patient care committee, grievance committee etc	❖ average length of stay ❖ complications rate ❖ readmission rate ❖ hospital infection rates ❖ death rates ❖ patient satisfaction ❖ hospital acquired infection rate ❖ referral rate

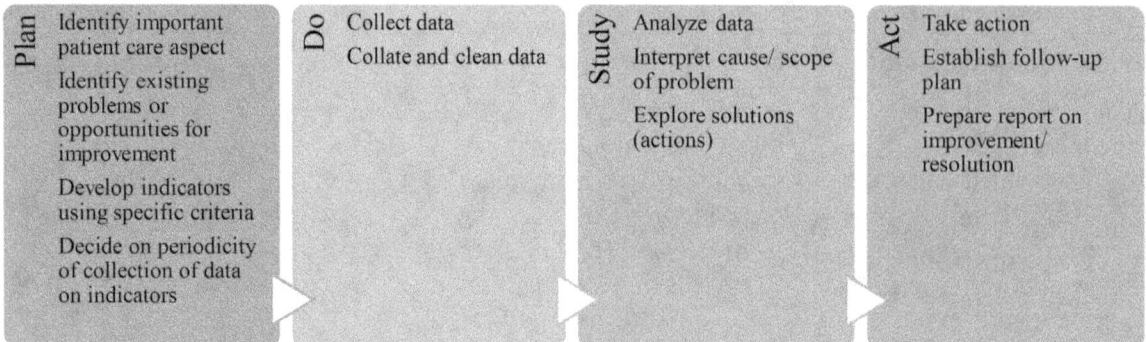

Figure 2: Steps of quality control in a hospital

Internal

- Comparison of similar processes and services within the organisation

Competitive

- Comparison with competitors in same sector

Functional

- Comparison with the best in the sector, but not direct competitor

Generic

- Comparison with other type of organisation having one or more similar process/dimension of performance

Figure 2: Types of Benchmarking

Chapter 13

	Revenue	Capital
Receipts	Recurring frequency	Non recurring frequency
	Received for rendering services or providing goods from recipient of such services/goods	Received to finance the fixed assets from owners or long-term loan providers or donors
	Helps to cover the day-to-day operational expenses	Helps to increase the capacity to service or produce more
	Shown in oncome statement under incomes	Shown in balance sheet under capital
Expenditure	Recurring frequency	Non recurring frequency
	Benefit obtained from such expenditure is for short term only	Benefit obtained from such expenditure is available for long term
	Incurred for day-to-day operational activities	Helps for increasing the existing capacity to service or produce more or add new capacity
	Shown in oncome statement under expenditure	Shown in balance sheet under Fixed Assets

	Cost Center	Revenue Center	Profit Center	Investment Center
What managers / supervisors manages	Cost only	Generates revenue	Earns profit. Incurs cost and generates revenue also.	Funds capex
Objective of responsibility center	Minimization of expenses	Maximization of revenues	Maximization of profits	Building capacity

Mission of Organisation and Performance Indicator to Refer to	Earning Profits	Serving Society
Main Performance Indicators	Financial	Non-financial
Additional Performance Indicator	Non-financial	Financial

Mission of Organisation and Performance Indicators	Earning Profit	Serving Society
Main Performance Measures	Operating cash flows Profits — gross and net Return on Investment (RoI) Profit Before Interest Tax (PBIT) Profit After Tax (PAT) Economic Value Added (EVA)	Patients attended/Day Patients attended/Doctor Percentage of Patients Treated Successfully
Additional Performance Measures	Percentage of Market Share Change in Percentage of Market Share Customer Satisfaction Rating Employee Satisfaction Rating	Excess of Income over Expenditure/Deficit Percentage of Increase In Donations/Funds Percentage of Reduction in Costs

CHAPTER 14

Classification of Leadership Based on		
Origin	Purpose	Nature
Executive Appointed	Intellectual	Authoritarian
Leader Appointed	Artistic	Democratic
Self-Appointed	Executive	Institutional
		Dominant
		Expert
		Persuasive

Chapter 15

Category	Classification
Yellow	(1) **Human Anatomical Waste**
	(2) **Animal Anatomical Waste**
	(3) **Soiled Waste**
	(4) **Discarded or Expired Medicine**
	(5) **Chemical Waste**
	(6) **Chemical Liquid Waste**
	(7) **Discarded linen, mattresses, beddings contaminated with blood or body fluid, routine mask and gown.**
	(8) **Microbiology, Biotechnology and other clinical laboratory waste (Pre-treated**
Red	Contaminated waste (recyclable)
White	Waste sharps including metals, needles, syringes with fixed needles
Blue	Broken or discarded and contaminated glass including medicine vials and ampoules except those contaminated with cytotoxic wastes.

Category	Colour and Type of Container for Collection
Yellow	Yellow coloured non-chlorinated plastic bags Chemical waste (yellow-e) should be stored in yellow container
Red	Red coloured non chlorinated plastic bags (having thickness equal to more than 50 µ) and containers
White	White coloured translucent, puncture proof, leak proof, temper proof containers
Blue	Puncture proof, leak proof boxes or containers with blue coloured marking

Category	Treatment
Yellow	No treatment of waste is required to be carried out at the healthcare facility except pre-treatment (sterilisation) of Yellow (h) category waste by autoclaving/microwaving or sterilise as per WHO Blue book 2014.
Red	Contaminated recyclable waste containing mainly plastics and rubber put in red coloured non chlorinated plastic bags and containers.
White	Collection in puncture proof, leak proof, tamper proof container ⟶ handover waste to CBWTF.
Blue (a) Glassware	Dispose of the empty glass bottles by handing over to CBWTF. The residual chemicals in glass bottle should be collected as chemical waste in yellow coloured container/bags and over to CBWTF as yellow (e) waste.
Blue (b)	Dispose of the waste by handing over to CBWTF. In case of no access to CBWTF, metallic body implants should be disinfected and later washed with detergent prior to sending/selling to metal recyclers.

CHAPTER 16

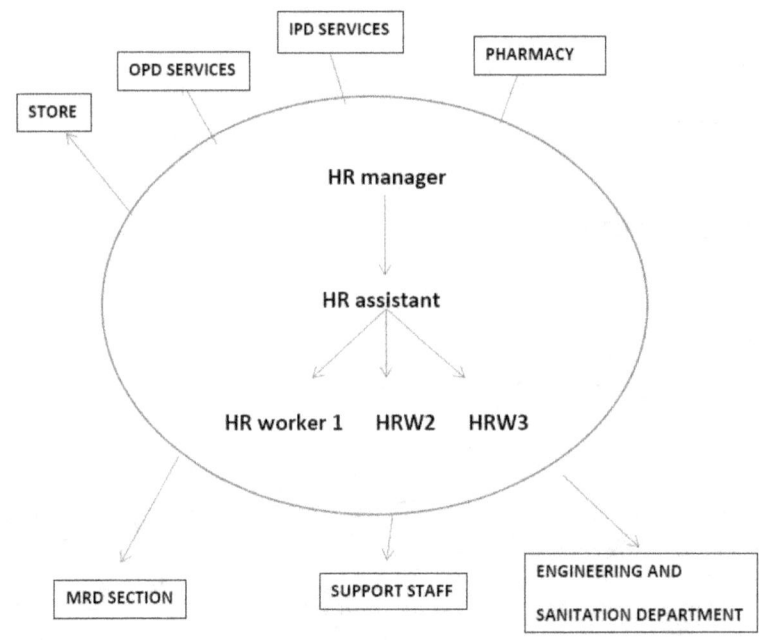

CHAPTER 17

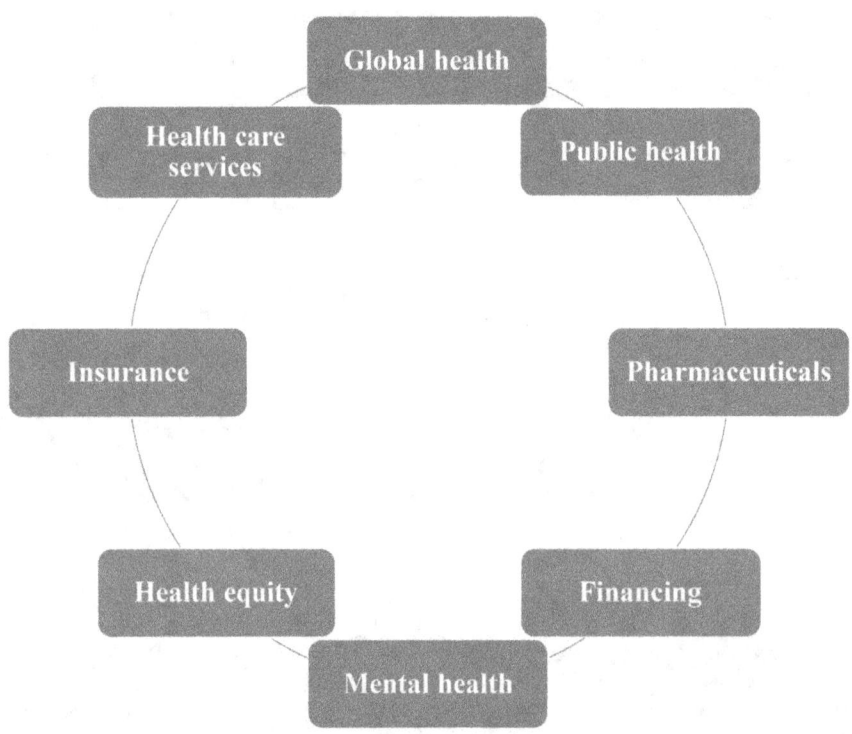

Chapter 18

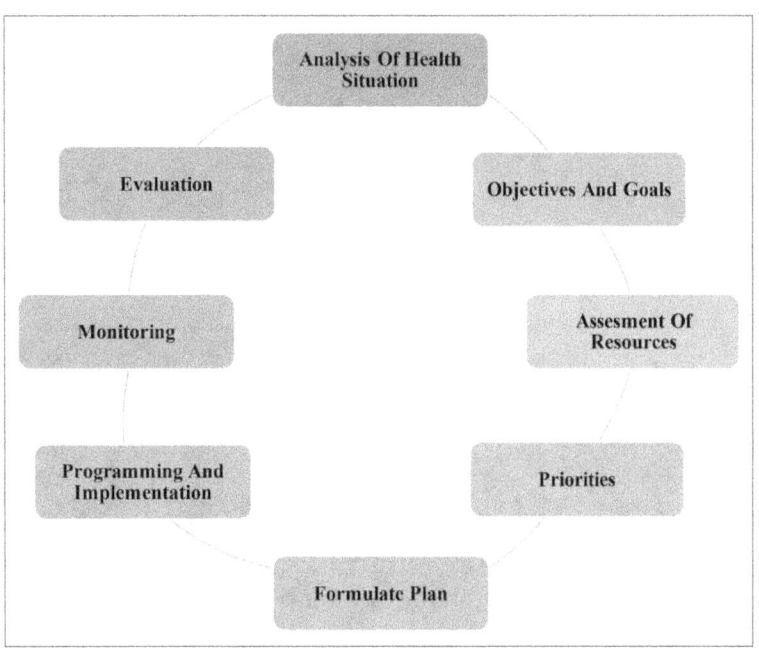

Chapter 19

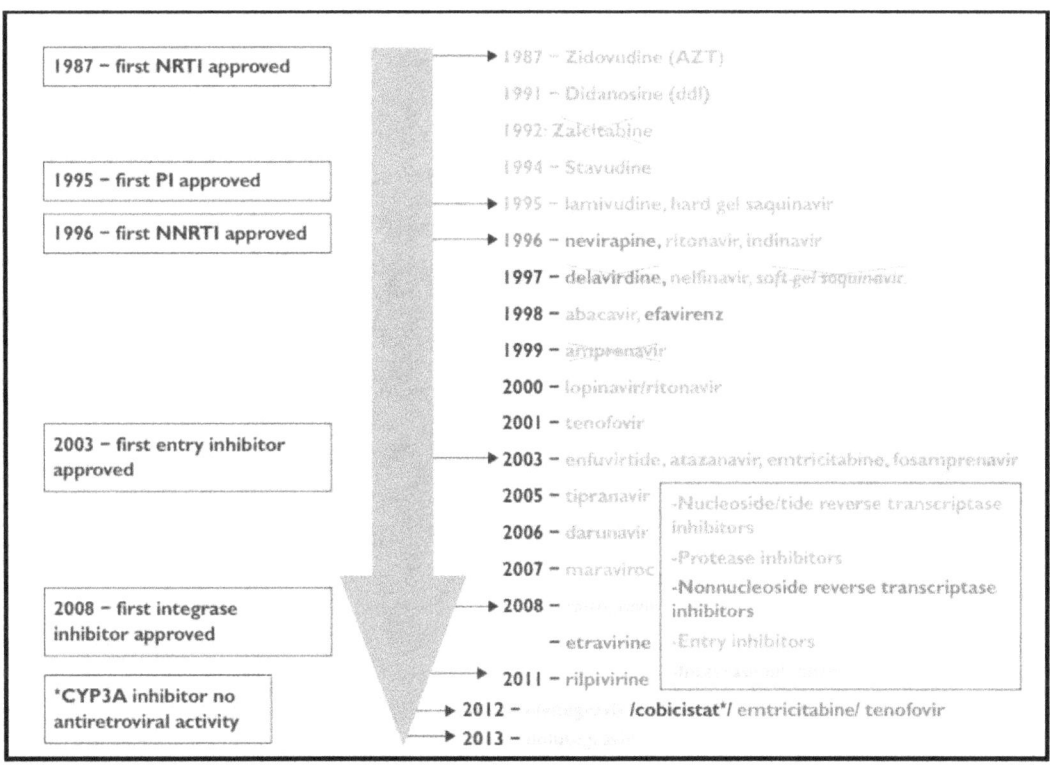

Figure 1: The time course of development ART drugs, highlighted according to the US Food and Drug Administration (FDA) approval date. Those that are no longer in use or available are illustrated with an 'X' through them

Table 1: Currently available antiretroviral drugs

Nucleoside Reverse Transcriptase Inhibitors (NsRTI)	Non Nucleoside Reverse Transcriptase Inhibitors (NNRTI)	Protease Inhibitors (PI)
• Zidovudine (AZT/ZDV)	• Nevirapine (NVP)	• Saquinavir (SQV)
• Stavudine (d4T)	• Efavirenz (EFV)	• Ritonavir (RTV)
• Lamivudine (3TC)	• Delavirdine (DLV)	• Nelfinavir (NFV)
• Abacavir (ABC)	• Rilpivirine (RPV)	• Amprenavir (APV)
• Didanosine (ddI)	• Etravirine (ETV)	• Indinavir (INV)
• Zalcitabine (ddC)	**Integrase Inhibitors**	• Lopinavir (LPV)
• Emtricitabine (FTC)	• Raltegravir (RGV)	• Fosamprenavir (FPV)
Nucleotide Reverse Transcriptase Inhibitors (NtRTI)	• Elvitegravir (EVG)	• Atazanavir (ATV)
	• Dolutegravir (DTG)	• Tipranavir (TPV)
• Tenofovir (TDF)		• Darunavir (DRV)
Fusion Inhibitors (FI)	**CCR5 Entry Inhibitor**	**Monoclonal Antibody**
• Enfuvirtide (T 20)	• Maraviroc	• Ibalizumab

Chapter 21

बांध / बहुगुणा बनाम बहुगुणा

बांध खतरा नहीं, जहां देखिए विकास ही लाए

बांध समर्थक

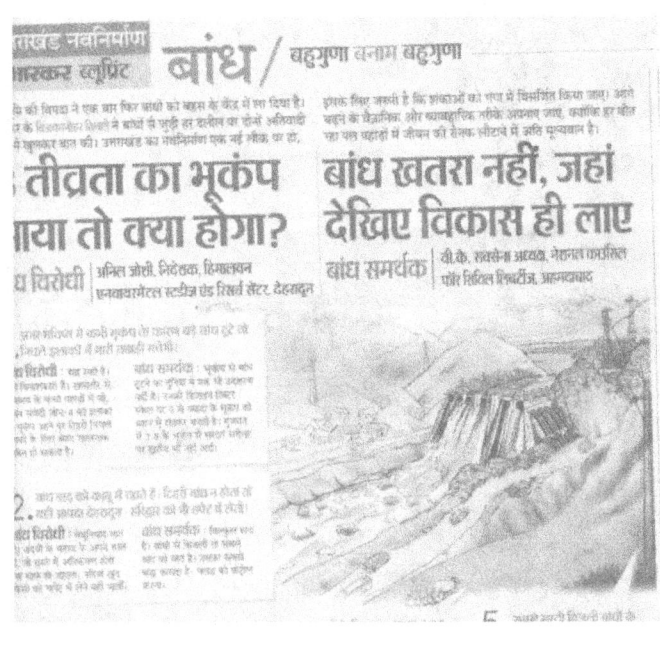

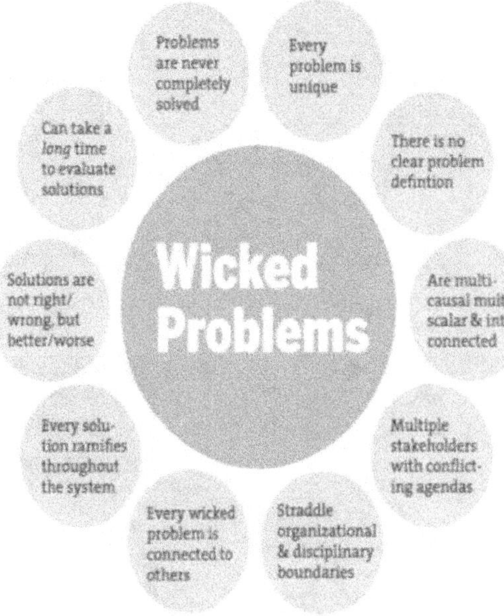

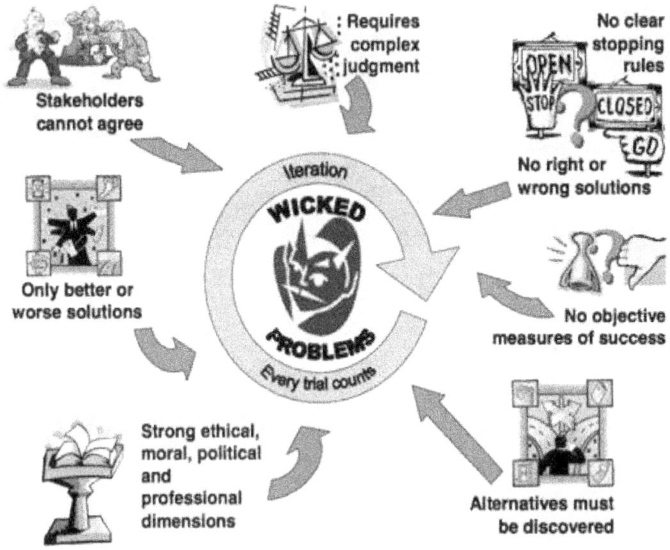

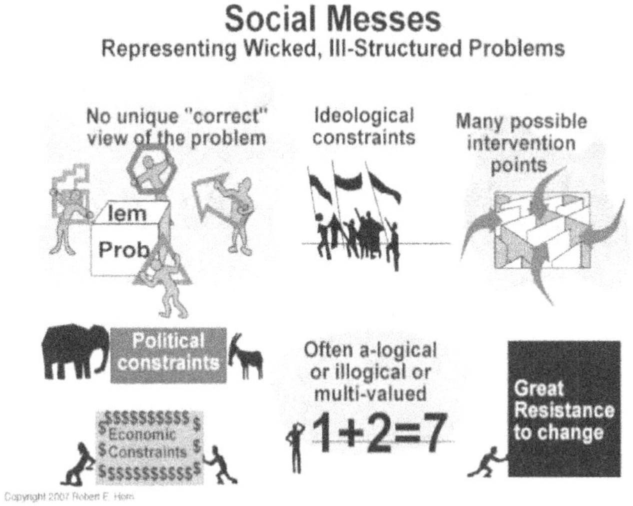

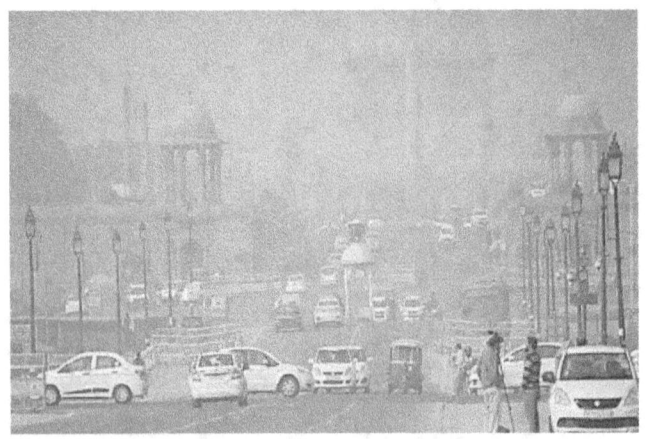

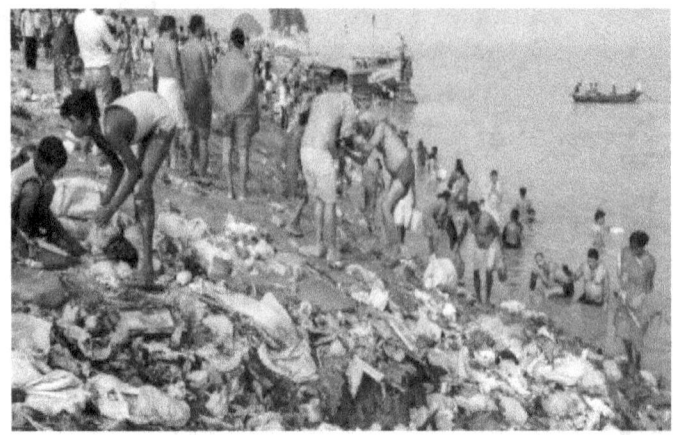

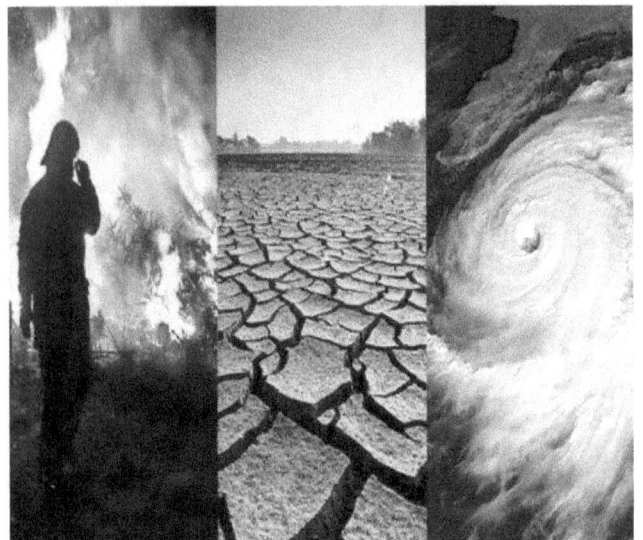

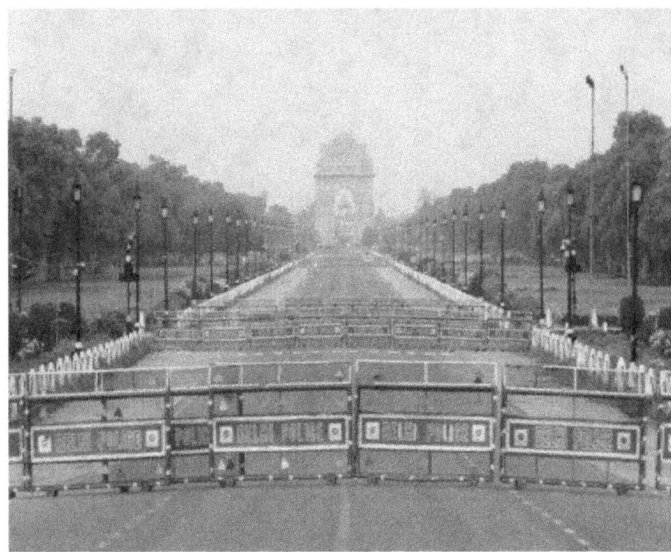

www.ingramcontent.com/pod-product-compliance
Lightning Source LLC
Chambersburg PA
CBHW081124170526
45165CB00008B/2534